SELF-ASSESSMENT IN
MEDICAL GENETICS

SELF-ASSESSMENT IN
MEDICAL GENETICS

J. M. CONNOR
MD, BSc, MRCP
*Wellcome Trust Senior Lecturer and
Honorary Consultant in Medical Genetics*

J. R. W. YATES
MA, MB, MRCP
*Consultant in Medical Genetics and
Honorary Clinical Lecturer*

*Both of the University of Glasgow and
Duncan Guthrie Institute of Medical Genetics,
Yorkhill, Glasgow*

BLACKWELL SCIENTIFIC PUBLICATIONS
OXFORD LONDON EDINBURGH
BOSTON PALO ALTO MELBOURNE

©1986 by
Blackwell Scientific Publications
Editorial offices:
Osney Mead, Oxford, OX2 OEL
8 John Street, London, WC1N 2ES
23 Ainslie Place, Edinburgh, EH3 6AJ
52 Beacon Street, Boston
    Massachusetts 02108, USA
667 Lytton Avenue, Palo Alto
    California 94301, USA
107 Barry Street, Carlton
    Victoria 3053, Australia

First published 1986

Set by Setrite Typesetters, Hong Kong
and printed and bound in Great
Britain by Clark Constable, Edinburgh

DISTRIBUTORS

USA
    Blackwell Mosby Book Distributors
    11830 Westline Industrial Drive
    St Louis, Missouri 63141

Canada
    Blackwell Mosby Book Distributors
    120 Melford Drive, Scarborough
    Ontario M1B 2X4

Australia
    Blackwell Scientific Publications
        (Australia) Pty Ltd
    107 Barry Street
    Carlton, Victoria 3053

British Library
Cataloguing in Publication Data

Connor, J. M.
    Self-assessment in medical genetics
    1. Medical Genetics
    I. Title.   II. Yates, J. R. W.
    616'-042   RB155

ISBN 0-632-01452-0

Contents

Preface

The growing importance of medical genetics in clinical practice reflects the decline in morbidity and mortality from other causes and advances in our understanding of the basic mechanisms of genetic disease. However, medical genetics is a recent inclusion in most undergraduate curricula and much of this new information lies scattered in journals and specialized texts. This book provides doctors with a means of updating their knowledge of medical genetics, particularly in preparation for examinations such as the MRCP and MRCOG, using a question and answer format.

More than 4000 genetic disorders are known, but most are rare and unlikely to be seen outside a specialist clinic. For this book 150 conditions have been chosen which illustrate recent advances, have treatable complications or are likely to be encountered in everyday practice or postgraduate examinations.

Whilst an elementary knowledge of genetics is assumed, basic principles are reviewed in the initial questions and a detailed glossary is provided.

Acknowledgements

We are most grateful to Professor Malcolm Ferguson-Smith for the clinical photographs used in questions 17, 18, 22, 24, 26, 33, 39, 52, 66, 84, 85, 86, 91, 92 96, 99, 108, 125 and 155. For permission to reproduce other figures thanks are due to Dr Nabeel Affara (question 8), Blackwell Scientific Publications (questions 2, 3, 4, 5, 16, 21, 27, 29, 33, 34, 38, 47, 48, 54, 62, 87 and 128), Dr John Dagg (question 112), Dr Kay MacDermot (question 111), Dr Heather May (questions 23, 65, 130, 133 and 134), Mr Peter Raine (question 64) and Dr Robin Winter (question 120). We are also grateful to Dr Elizabeth Boyd for preparing the karyotypes and to Miss Aileen Robertson for typing the manuscript.

We also wish to thank Professor Malcolm Ferguson-Smith, Dr David Gilmore, Dr Mary King and Dr John Tolmie for their valuable comments on the manuscript.

Basic Principles

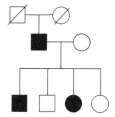

1 This is a typical autosomal dominant pedigree drawn using the conventional symbols given below.

   a What are the characteristic features of autosomal dominant inheritance?

   b Draw a simple pedigree to illustrate the features of autosomal recessive inheritance.

   c Draw a simple pedigree to illustrate the features of X-linked recessive inheritance.

Pedigree symbols

☐   Normal male   ○   Normal female

■   Affected male   ●   Affected female

◧ ◐   Autosomal recessive carriers (heterozygotes)

⊙   X-linked carrier female

⊠   Deceased male   Abortion

☐—○   Marriage   ☐═○   Consanguineous marriage

Twins   Monozygotic twins

↗   Indicates proband (syn. index case, propositus)

C   Indicates consultand (the individual seeking advice)

1   a   Autosomal dominant inheritance. Heterozygotes manifest the
disorder. On average half of their offspring inherit the disease
gene, males and females being equally at risk. The severity of
the disease may vary from one individual to another (variable
expression) and in some dominant conditions not all
heterozygotes develop the disorder (incomplete penetrance).
Autosomal dominant diseases may arise as the result of a new
mutation, as appears to be the case in the family shown. An
alternative explanation is that one of the grandparents carried
the disease gene but did not manifest the condition because of
non-penetrance or death before symptoms developed in the
case of late onset disorders.

   b   Autosomal recessive inheritance

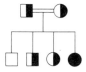

Homozygotes manifest the disorder but heterozygotes (carriers)
do not. Both parents must be carriers and on average a quarter
of their offspring will be affected. Males and females are equally
at risk. Consanguinity may be responsible for bringing together
carriers of the same disorder, particularly if the condition is
rare, and is indicated by double lines between them.

   c   X-linked recessive inheritance.

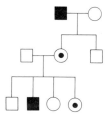

Hemizygous males manifest the disease whilst heterozygous
females (carriers) are affected only mildly or not at all. The
daughters of an affected male inherit his X chromosome bearing
the disease gene and must all be carriers, whereas the sons
receive his Y chromosome and cannot inherit the disorder. Male
to male transmission excludes X-linked inheritance. On
average, half the sons of a carrier female will be healthy and half
will be affected, half of her daughters will be carriers. X-linked
recessive disorders can arise as the result of a new mutation.

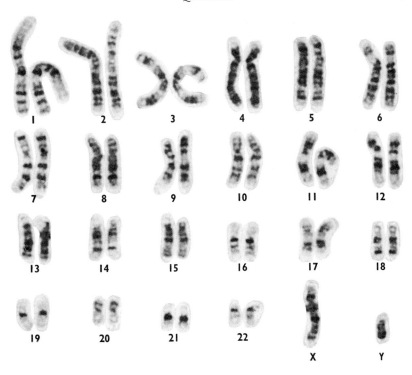

2 a What does this picture show?
   b Which stage of cell division does this represent?
   c What is the significance of the banding?
   d Which tissues are suitable for this type of analysis?

2 **Standard karyotype**
  a A routine G (Giemsa) banded karyotype from a normal male.
  b Mitotic cell division is arrested at metaphase by colchicine.
  c The banding reflects differential chromosomal condensation. About 300 alternating light and dark bands are present and each chromosome pair can be distinguished by its characteristic banding pattern.
  d Chromosomes are most conveniently studied in peripheral blood lymphocytes from a heparinized blood sample. Cultured skin fibroblasts, bone marrow, tumour tissue, amniotic fluid cells and chorionic villi can also be used.

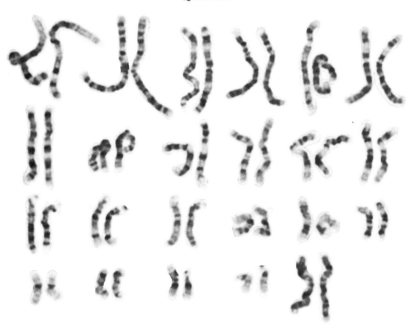

3 a What does this picture show?
   b What are the advantages of this type of preparation?
   c What is the smallest visible addition or deletion from a
      chromosome?
   d Why are chromosomes not routinely analysed in this way?

4 **This is an epithelial cell nucleus from a buccal smear.**
   a What feature does this cell nucleus show?
   b What is the sex of this individual?
   c Would all the nuclei on the smear show this feature?

3 **Prometaphase karyotype**
   a A G-banded karyotype from a normal female. The chromosomes
      are less condensed than in the previous karyotype because
      mitosis has been arrested at prometaphase (see footnote).
   b In a prometaphase spread up to 1000 bands can be identified
      and the increased resolution may reveal deletions or
      rearrangements not visible using routine metaphase
      preparations.
   c The smallest visible change in a chromosome is about one band
      which represents 50—100 genes based on an estimated total
      number of 50 000—100 000 genes in man.
   d Prometaphase banding is technically complicated and time
      consuming.

4 **Barr body**
   a There is a densely stained chromatin mass adjacent to the
      nuclear membrane known as the Barr body or X-chromatin.
   b Every cell maintains one activated X chromosome. Any
      additional X chromosomes are inactivated and appear as Barr
      bodies. The number of X chromosomes is therefore one more
      than the number of Barr bodies per cell and a Barr body is not
      seen in males. In this case there is one Barr body and hence two
      X chromosomes are present. The individual is likely to be
      female but if phenotypically male could have Klinefelter
      syndrome (47, XXY).
   c X-chromatin is only visible during certain stages of the cell
      cycle and about 30% of nuclei on a buccal smear from a normal
      female show a Barr body.

Footnote: Currently karyotypes used in the data interpretation section of MRCP
       do not have numbers against the chromosomes. Hence some karyo-
       types are presented in this form.

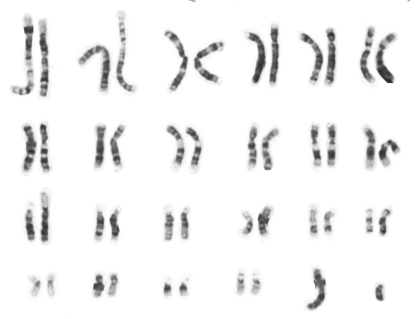

5 **This is a chromosome preparation from a healthy male.**
   a What is the abnormality?
   b What is the significance of this abnormality?
   c How is it inherited?

6 **Each strand of DNA has a sugar-phosphate backbone with projecting bases.**
   a What types of bases occur in DNA?
   b How do bases pair with the complementary strand of DNA?
   c How many bases constitute an aminoacid codon?

5   **Chromosome variation**
   a   One homologue of chromosome 13 has an elongated short arm.
   b   This short arm contains unimportant DNA and this is a
       harmless chromosome variant or heteromorphism. Such minor
       heritable differences are present in at least 30% of the
       population and the commonest relates to the length of the long
       arm of the Y chromosome.
   c   On average this variant will be transmitted unchanged to half of
       his offspring.

6   **DNA structure**
   a   There are two purine bases called adenine (A) and guanine (G)
       and two pyrimidine bases called thymine (T) and cytosine (C).
   b   G always pairs with C and A with T.
   c   An aminoacid codon consists of three bases. As each base in the
       triplet may be any of the four types of nucleotide (A,G,C,T) this
       results in 64 possible codons. Most aminoacids have more than
       one codon and some codons signal chain termination.

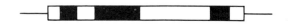

7   **This is a diagram of a typical human gene.**
   a   How large in terms of base pairs of DNA are human genes?
   b   What do the light and dark areas represent?
   c   What are the steps involved in the production of a protein from
       a gene?
   d   How much of the chromosomal DNA is in the form of
       functioning genes?

7 Gene structure and function

a The example shown is the β globin gene which is 1600 base pairs in length. Human genes so far studied have ranged from 1000–180 000 base pairs (1–180 kilobases or kb). This is much larger than predicted from their protein products because of intervening sequences and post-translational modifications.

b The dark areas (known as exons) are coding sequences for aminoacids. The light areas (known as intervening sequences or introns) are non-coding sequences of unkown function.

c An RNA copy of the entire gene is made on the DNA template (transcription). This messenger RNA is then modified by excision (splicing) of the RNA corresponding to the introns. The mature messenger RNA is translated into its protein product by ribosomes in the cytoplasm. The initial polypeptide may undergo post-translational modifications to form the final product. An abnormal protein can result from faults at any level in this process.

d There are an estimated 50 000–100 000 genes in man. If the average gene is 3 kilobases in length then this probably only accounts for 10% of the total DNA. Some of the remainder is involved in the regulation of gene expression but the function of the rest (perhaps 40% of the total DNA) is unknown.

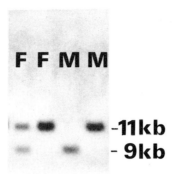

8   This is an autoradiograph demonstrating a restriction fragment
    length polymorphism (RFLP) on the X chromosome detected with
    the DNA probe 754. Four individuals have been tested, two
    females and two males.
    a   What is the origin of this pattern?
    b   Are all the possible fragment patterns shown?

8   Restriction fragment length polymorphism

a Restriction enzymes (endonucleases) cut DNA in a sequence
specific manner. For example, the enzyme Pst I cuts the DNA
wherever the following sequence occurs:

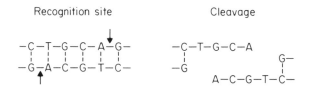

This is used to demonstrate differences in DNA sequence
between individuals (polymorphism). On the X chromosome in
the vicinity of the DNA probe 754 two situations can be found:

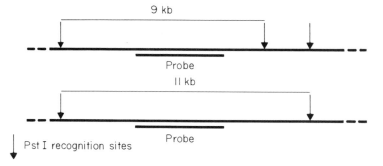

The upper chromosome shows the less common arrangement
(36%) with Pst I recognition sites either side of the probe at
points 9000 base pairs apart so that digestion with this enzyme
yields a 9 kb fragment. The lower chromosome shows the more
common arrangement (64%). There is a different DNA sequence
at the position of the second site, which need only involve a
change in a single base pair, and the recognition site is
abolished. The enzyme cuts at another site further away and the
resulting fragment is 11 000 base pairs long (11 kb).

The fragments are separated by gel electrophoresis and
identified from amongst the hundreds of thousands of other
fragments present by means of the radiolabelled probe 754
which hybridizes to its complementary DNA sequences.

b No. Males have one X chromosome and depending on which
DNA sequence is present will show either an 11 kb or a 9 kb
fragment. Females have two X chromosomes which can yield
two 11 kb fragments, one 11 kb and one 9 kb fragment or two
9 kb fragments. The last of these patterns is not shown.

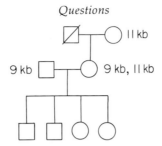

9   This family has been partially studied with the DNA probe 754 to
     show the restriction fragment length polymorphism described in
     the previous question.
     a   What fragment pattern must have been present in the
          grandfather?
     b   What fragment patterns are possible in the grandchildren?

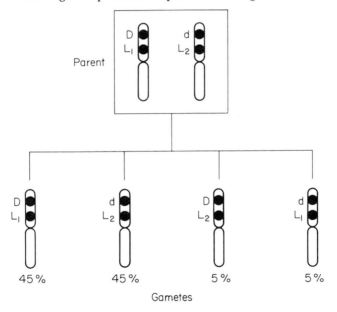

10   This is a diagram of a disease and marker locus on the same
      chromosome showing genetic linkage. The disease is autosomal
      dominant and caused by the allele D whilst the corresponding
      normal allele is d. The marker is a restriction fragment length
      polymorphism with fragments of length L_1 and L_2. Four types of
      gamete are possible and are produced in the proportions shown.
      a   What is genetic linkage?
      b   What is the recombination fraction?
      c   Are loci on the same chromosome always linked?
      d   What is the phase in the parent?

9   Restriction fragment length polymorphism

   a   The grandfather must have had a 9 kb restriction fragment. His
         daughter is heterozygous with 9 kb and 11 kb fragments and
         since her mother is homozygous with both X chromosomes
         yielding the 11 kb fragment it follows that the 9 kb fragment
         must have come from her father.

   b   Depending on which pattern they inherit with the X
         chromosome from their mother, the boys will either show a
         9 kb or 11 kb fragment. The girls all receive a 9 kb fragment on
         the X chromosome inherited from their father, and depending
         on which pattern they inherit from their mother will either
         show two 9 kb fragments or one 9 kb and one 11 kb fragment.

10   Genetic linkage

   a   According to Mendel, genes for different traits are inherited
         independently of one another. This holds true for loci on
         different chromosomes, but not for neighbouring loci on the
         same chromosome. In this situation the tendency for genes to
         segregate together is called genetic linkage. In the example
         above, 90% of the gametes are DL_1 or dL_2, retaining the same
         relationship between disease and marker alleles as in the parent
         and representing a striking departure from independent
         assortment.

   b   Gametes of type dL_1 and DL_2 are the result of crossing-over
         (recombination) at meiosis and the recombination fraction is
         the fraction of gametes which are recombinants, in this case
         1/10 th (10%). If the loci are very close together on the same
         chromosome, crossing-over will be rare and the recombination
         fraction approaches zero.

   c   No. When loci are far apart on the same chromosome, crossing-
         over abolishes any tendency for alleles to segregate together and
         in effect there is independent assortment. All four types of
         gamete are equally likely and the recombination fraction is ½
         (50%).

   d   Phase refers to the arrangement of the disease and marker
         alleles. In this case the parent has D and L_1 on one chromosome,
         d and L_2 on the other. The alternative possibility would be D
         and L_2 on one chromosome, d and L_1 on the other. In both cases
         the restriction fragment pattern is $L_1 L_2$ and the phase can only
         be deduced by studying other family members.

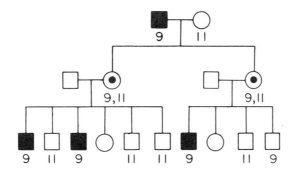

11 This family shows X-linked recessive inheritance of Becker muscular dystrophy. The family has been studied with the DNA probe 754 to show the restriction fragment length polymorphism described previously.

   a What is the phase in the female carriers in the second generation?

   b What is the recombination fraction?

   c Does this family provide evidence for linkage between Becker muscular dystrophy and this DNA marker?

11   Genetic linkage

  a   The Becker muscular dystrophy gene and 9 kb restriction
        fragment are together on the X chromosome inherited from
        their affected father. The normal gene at the Becker locus and
        the 11 kb fragment are on the other X chromosome inherited
        from the mother.

  b   In the third generation all three males with Becker muscular
        dystrophy show the 9 kb fragment and four of the five
        unaffected males have the 11 kb fragment retaining the
        relationship between disease and marker alleles present in their
        mother. The youngest male is the only recombinant, having
        inherited the 9 kb fragment but not the disease. The
        recombination fraction is therefore one eighth.

  c   The findings in this family provide support for linkage between
        Becker muscular dystrophy and this DNA marker (but do not in
        themselves reach statistical significance). Extensive family
        studies have confirmed this linkage and the estimated
        recombination fraction is 10%.

        This DNA marker is also linked to Duchenne muscular
        dystrophy with a similar recombination fraction. Other linkage
        data confirm that the Duchenne and Becker muscular dystrophy
        loci are close together on the short arm of the X chromosome,
        and the striking similarities in their phenotype supports the
        hypothesis that they result from different alleles at the same
        locus. This is one of several linked DNA markers which offer
        the prospect of carrier detection and prenatal diagnosis for
        these disorders.

Specific Disorders

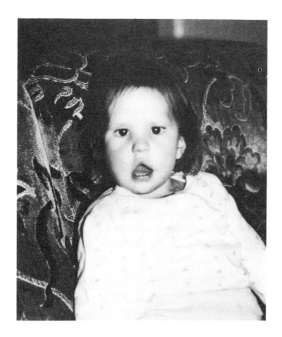

12 **This child required respiratory support in the newborn period. She was extremely hypotonic and had to be fed by nasogastric tube for several months. She is still hypotonic and her development is significantly delayed.**

  a What is the likely diagnosis?
  b Are other individuals in the family likely to show evidence of this disorder?
  c What is the recurrence risk?
  d Is prenatal diagnosis available?

12   Myotonic dystrophy

a This child has the characteristic tent-shaped upper lip seen in congenital myotonic dystrophy due to the associated facial weakness.

b This is an autosomal dominant disorder. The typical adult presenting with myotonic dystrophy has myotonia of grip, an expressionless face, ptosis and wasting and weakness of sternomastoids and distal upper and lower limb musculature. There may be cataracts and males show frontal baldness and testicular atrophy. There is, however, a wide range of expression and a substantial minority of gene carriers are asymptomatic and can only be detected by careful clinical examination backed up by electromyography and slit lamp examination for lens opacities.

   In this family the child's mother was undiagnosed but had experienced difficulty relaxing her grip for several years. She had typical myopathic facies. Her mother and a sister were found to be asymptomatic carriers.

c Congenital myotonic dystrophy only occurs in children who inherit the mutant gene from their mother. It can manifest as stillbirth or severe neonatal illness with a substantial mortality. Many of the survivors are mentally handicapped. In a subsequent pregnancy the baby has a 50% chance of inheriting the myotonic dystrophy gene. For women who have already had children with congenital myotonic dystrophy, as in this case, the risk of another child with *neonatal* disease is 30%, substantially higher than the 6% risk for the mothers who have not had congenitally affected offspring.

d The locus for myotonic dystrophy is on chromosome 19. In the past prenatal diagnosis has been possible in only a minority of families by linkage to the secretor locus. Linked DNA markers are now becoming available for prenatal diagnosis and detection of asymptomatic gene carriers.

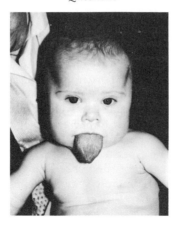

13 a What is the likely diagnosis?
    b What other features may be present?
    c What is the prognosis?
    d What is the recurrence risk?
    e What is the connection with chromosome 11?

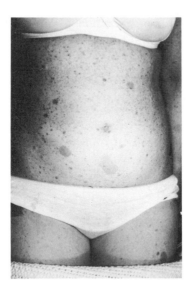

14 a What is the diagnosis?
    b What are the clinical features?
    c What complications may occur?
    d What is the mode of inheritance?
    e Is prenatal diagnosis available?

13   Beckwith—Wiedemann syndrome
  a   Macroglossia suggests the Beckwith—Wiedemann syndrome.
  b   High birth weight with large kidneys, liver and pancreas, exomphalos, ear lobe grooves, pits on the posterior rim of the ear pinna and occasionally hemihypertrophy. Neonatal hypoglycaemia with elevated plasma insulin levels is common.
  c   Neoplasia, especially Wilms tumour, occurs in 5% of cases. Mental retardation is occasionally present, especially if hypoglycaemia was inadequately treated.
  d   The recurrence risk is usually low but some familial cases have occurred with a pattern suggesting autosomal dominant inheritance with very variable expression. Prenatal diagnosis has been achieved by ultrasound scanning to show exomphalos, renal enlargement and macroglossia.
  e   A small duplication of band 11p15 has been found in a few patients.

14   Neurofibromatosis
  a   These are the typical skin lesions of neurofibromatosis.
  b   Multiple *cafe-au-lait* spots (at least five spots greater than 1.5 cm in diameter), axillary freckling (Crowe's sign) and multiple neurofibromata which usually appear in later childhood or adolescence. Cutaneous neurofibromas usually take the form of soft pedunculated masses. Neurofibromas attached to peripheral nerves are palpable as subcutaneous nodules. Lesions of the iris (Lisch nodules) and retinal phakomata may be present. Mild mental retardation is not infrequent.
  c   Neurological impairment due to neurofibromas forming on cranial nerves (especially acoustic neuromas) and spinal nerve roots. Neural tumours (optic nerve glioma, meningioma, phaeochromocytoma). Sarcomatous change in neurofibromas. Systemic hypertension.
  d   Autosomal dominant. About 50% of cases are new mutations but a careful family history and examination of immediate family members is essential before concluding that a patient represents a new mutation.
  e   Prenatal diagnosis is not possible.

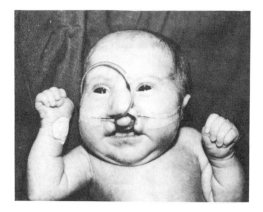

15 **This newborn is small for gestational age and has a ventricular septal defect.**
  a What is the likely diagnosis?
  b What other clinical features may be present?
  c What is the prognosis?
  d What is the recurrence risk?

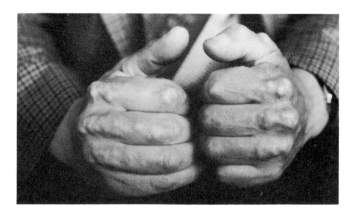

16 **This man's father and brother died suddenly in middle age.**
  a What is the diagnosis?
  b How may this diagnosis be confirmed?
  c What is the basic defect and how is this inherited?
  d What is the prognosis?

15 Trisomy 13

a Bilateral cleft lip and palate, microphthalmia with slanting palpebral fissures, low set ears, flexed fingers and congenital heart disease in a small for gestational age neonate suggests trisomy 13.

b Hypotelorism reflecting underlying holoprosencephaly, colobomas, scalp defects, polydactyly, prominent heels, cystic renal dysplasia and cryptorchidism in males.

c These infants show profound developmental delay and failure to thrive. Congenital heart disease is usual and 50% die within one month.

d The incidence is 1 in 5000 live births. The recurrence risk in young mothers is not established but by analogy with trisomy 21 may be as high as 1.5%. In women over 35 years of age this is exceeded by the increasing risk of chromosome abnormalities in older mothers. In cases of trisomy 13 phenotype due to a translocation involving chromosome 13 the parents need karyotyping to exclude a balanced translocation.

16 Familial hypercholesterolaemia

a The combination of tendon xanthomata and a family history of sudden death in middle age suggests familial hypercholesterolaemia.

b A fasting lipid profile shows elevated total cholesterol due to an increase in low density lipoprotein. Other lipoproteins and lipids are relatively normal.

c The basic defect is a deficiency of a specific cell surface receptor responsible for the uptake of low density lipoprotein. The condition is inherited as an autosomal dominant trait and the locus in on chromosome 19. One in 500 of the general population carry this mutant gene. If both parents are affected there is a 1 in 4 risk of a child homozygous for the disease (two copies of the mutant allele) who would die of coronary heart disease in childhood.

d 50% of heterozygous affected males die from coronary heart disease by 60 years of age. Drugs such as cholestyramine and dietary measures to reduce serum cholesterol may be beneficial.

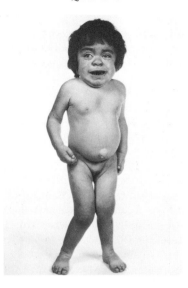

17 a What is the likely diagnosis?
    b What are the features of this condition?
    c How would this diagnosis be confirmed?
    d What is the mode of inheritance?
    e Is prenatal diagnosis available?

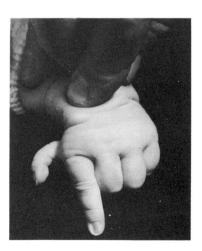

18 **This child has an atrial septal defect.**
    a What is the diagnosis?
    b What are the features of this condition?
    c What is the mode of inheritance?

17 Hurler syndrome

  a The large head, thick eyebrows, depressed nasal bridge, coarse
       facial features and protuberant abdomen with umbilical hernia
       are typical of Hurler syndrome (Mucopolysaccharidosis type
       IH).
  b Coarsening of facial features, corneal clouding, joint stiffness,
       kyphoscoliosis and hepatosplenomegaly with onset in infancy.
       Short stature and intellectual deterioration become apparent by
       2−3 years of age. Enlarged head, thick lips, large tongue, peg-
       like teeth, joint contractures, hirsutism and progressive
       deafness. Death by 10 years of age from pneumonia or cardiac
       failure is usual.
  c This is a storage disorder in which mucopolysaccharide
       accumulates in the tissues because of deficiency of the
       lysosomal enzyme alpha-iduronidase. The diagnosis can be
       confirmed by assay of this enzyme in leucocytes or cultured
       skin fibroblasts. The urine contains excess mucopolysaccharide
       (dermatan and heparan sulphate). X-rays show dysostosis
       multiplex.
  d Autosomal recessive. Hunter syndrome (MPS II) has somewhat
       similar clinical features but is X-linked recessive so that only
       males are affected.
  e Prenatal diagnosis is possible by two-dimensional
       electrophoresis of glycosaminoglycans (GAGs) in amniotic fluid
       and by specific enzyme assay in cultured amniotic fluid cells or
       chorionic villi.

18 Holt−Oram syndrome

  a A small distally placed triphalangeal thumb and congenital
       heart disease are characteristic of the Holt−Oram syndrome
       (Heart−hand syndrome).
  b The upper limb defect can range from a radiological
       abnormality of a clinically normal hand to phocomelia.
       Hypoplastic, triphalangeal or absent thumbs are the commonest
       finding. The lower limbs are normal. Secundum atrial septal
       defect is the characteristic cardiac anomaly but ventricular
       septal defect, patent ductus arteriosus and numerous other
       defects have been described.
  c Autosomal dominant with very variable expression.

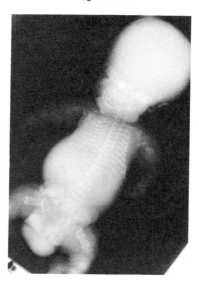

19 This is the x-ray of a stillborn male whose parents are healthy. Their previous pregnancy had resulted in a stillborn male with shortened deformed limbs.
  a What is the diagnosis?
  b What is the mode of inheritance?
  c Is prenatal diagnosis possible?

20 A non-consanguinous couple request counselling after the death of their son from *Pneumocystis carinii* pneumonia at 6 months of age. He had been underweight with a history of persistent oral thrush (monilia) and chronic diarrhoea. He had a total white cell count of 7.0×10^9/l with 70% neutrophils, 15% eosinophils, 10% lymphocytes and 5% monocytes. Immunoglobin levels were well below the normal range. A previous son also failed to thrive and died from chickenpox in early childhood.
  a What diagnosis is likely?
  b Are any tests helpful on the parents?
  c How is this condition inherited?
  d Is prenatal diagnosis possible?

19 Osteogenesis imperfecta

a The X-ray shows multiple fractures with shortening and deformation of the involved bones characteristic of osteogenesis imperfecta congenita (OIC). Hypophosphatasia can also cause defective ossification *in utero* with fractures but the radiological appearances differ from OIC and can be further excluded by the presence of normal levels of alkaline phosphatase in blood or skin fibroblasts.

b Overall the incidence of OIC is about 1 in 50 000 total births and the empiric recurrence risk after a sporadic case is 3%. This risk encompasses a small number of autosomal recessive cases and the majority of families where the condition is due to a new mutation with a negligible recurrence risk. In this family with two affected sibs autosomal recessive inheritance is likely with a 1 in 4 recurrence risk.

c Serial ultrasound scanning during the second trimester can demonstrate the defective ossification and limb shortening and angulation.

20 a Severe combined immunodeficiency

b In about 20% of patients with severe combined immunodeficiency (SCID) there is a reduced level of the enzyme adenosine deaminase (ADA) which can be assayed in red blood cells. Parents of these children have half the normal levels of this enzyme.

c SCID shows genetic heterogeneity with autosomal recessive and X-linked recessive types. The ADA deficient type is autosomal recessive and if the parents show carrier levels of this enzyme the recurrence risk would be 1 in 4 and independent of the sex of the child.

d In families with ADA deficiency prenatal diagnosis is possible by measurement of this enzyme in amniotic fluid cells or chorionic villi. In the remainder fetal blood sampling is required to show absence of T and B lymphocyte surface markers.

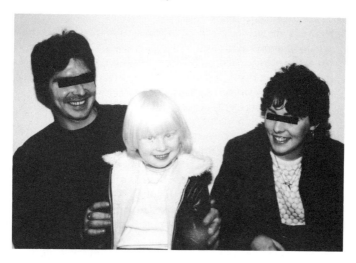

21 **a** What is the diagnosis?
   b What are the two common forms of this disorder?
   c What is the prognosis?
   d What is the risk of recurrence in subsequent children?
   e What is the risk to the girl's offspring?

21 Oculocutaneous albinism

  a The striking lack of pigment of the skin and hair are typical of oculocutaneous albinism.

  b There are several types of albinism but the commonest forms are tyrosinase positive and tyrosinase negative. In the latter, absence of tyrosinase can be demonstrated in hair bulbs and pigment is completely lacking. The skin is pink-red and there is a striking red reflex from the fundus. Nystagmus and photophobia are severe and visual acuity is impaired. In tyrosinase positive albinos a small amount of pigment may accumulate with age, resulting in some improvement in visual acuity; nystagmus and photophobia are less severe.

  c Visual acuity is impaired especially in tyrosinase negative individuals. There is an increased susceptibility to skin cancer.

  d Albinism is an autosomal recessive trait with a 1 in 4 recurrence risk.

  e Since this girl is homozygous for the mutant allele all of her offspring will be carriers. She could only have affected children if she was married to a carrier *for the same type* of albinism. (Tyrosinase positive and tyrosinase negative albinism both have a carrier frequency of 1 in 100).

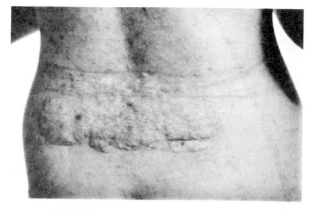

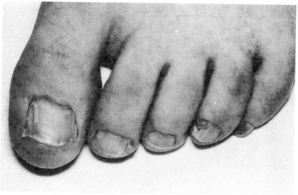

22 **This girl has epilepsy. Her parents are both healthy.**
   a What is the diagnosis?
   b What other features should be looked for?
   c What is the prognosis?
   d What is the recurrence risk?

22   Tuberous sclerosis

   a   A shagreen patch and subungual fibroma are characteristic
       lesions of tuberous sclerosis.

   b   Adenoma sebaceum (facial angiofibromas which develop in late
       childhood or adolescence in about 80% of patients),
       depigmented 'ash leaf' skin patches (80%), whitish raised
       lesions on the retina (phakomas), pitted dental enamel and
       intracranial calcification (after infancy).

   c   Epilepsy (90%) and mental retardation (60%) are the most
       serious manifestations. Benign tumours may occur in various
       organs, epecially the kidneys. Cardiac rhabdomyoma is a rare
       but important complication causing heart failure and
       arrhythmias. Prognosis is very variable. Some patients are
       asymptomatic and others require institutional care. Premature
       death may result from status epilepticus, brain tumour or renal
       failure.

   d   Tuberous sclerosis is an autosomal dominant disorder, but at
       least two-thirds of cases are new mutations. This may well be
       the situation in this family, since the parents are healthy. But
       before concluding that the risk to subsequent children is very
       small, both parents should be carefully examined, including
       inspection of the skin under ultraviolet light for depigmented
       patches, and cranial CT scan should be considered.
          The risk to the offspring of the affected girl is 1 in 2.

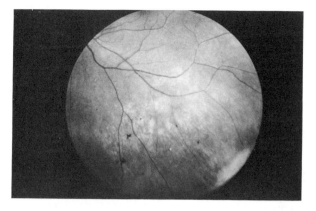

23 **This woman's brother was registered blind in his twenties.**
   a What is the diagnosis?
   b What is the mode of inheritance?

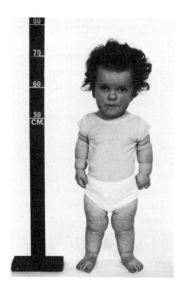

24 **This is a two-year-old girl. Her parents are of normal stature.**
   a What is the likely diagnosis?
   b How could this diagnosis be confirmed?
   c What is the prognosis?
   d What is the recurrence risk?

23 a Retinitis pigmentosa.

   b Transmission of retinitis pigmentosa (RP) may be autosomal
        dominant, autosomal recessive or X-linked recessive and a
        minority of cases are non-genetic. The mode of inheritance may
        be clear if several family members are affected. Otherwise it is
        essential to evaluate close relatives by ophthalmological
        examination and retinal function tests to detect asymptomatic
        cases. This is particularly likely in the mild autosomal dominant
        type of RP where penetrance is incomplete and in female
        carriers of X-linked recessive RP who are seldom symptomatic
        but usually show characteristic fundal changes by early adult
        life.
            In this case, X-linked retinitis pigmentosa is the most likely
        diagnosis and other at risk female relatives should be examined.
        Linked DNA markers are under evaluation for carrier detection
        and prenatal diagnosis in X-linked retinitis pigmentosa.

24 Achondroplasia

   a The combination of short stature with proximal (rhizomelic)
        limb shortening, a prominent forehead and a depressed nasal
        bridge suggests achondroplasia.

   b Skeletal survey shows characteristic changes including caudal
        narrowing of the lumbar interpedicular distances.

   c Intelligence and lifespan are normal but short stature is
        invariable (adult males about 132 cm and adult females about
        125 cm). Backache is common but cord compression is rare.
        Hydrocephalus is rare but often misdiagnosed because the skull
        base is short and the vault therefore enlarges to accommodate a
        normal sized brain. Normal growth charts for achondroplastic
        children are available.

   d This is an autosomal dominant trait with full penetrance so that
        the risk to this girl's offspring will be 1 in 2. Since the parents
        are of normal stature this child must be the result of a new
        mutation. The risk of recurrence in subsequent children is
        therefore negligible.

25 **A 30-year-old man with panacinar emphysema requests advice about the risks to his offspring. His sister died in the newborn period with obstructive jaundice.**
   a What diagnosis is suggested?
   b How may this be confirmed?
   c What is the prognosis?
   d What is the risk to his offspring?

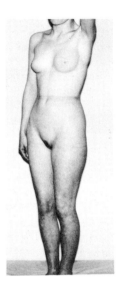

26 **This patient presented with primary amenorrhoea and has normal female external genitalia, a short blind-ending vagina and absent uterus. Karyotype is 46 XY.**
   a What is the likely diagnosis?
   b What other physical findings would support this diagnosis?
   c What is the underlying defect?
   d How is this condition inherited?
   e What is the prognosis?

25 a Alpha-1-antitrypsin deficiency.
    b Assay will confirm reduced protease inhibitor activity and
        isoelectric focusing shows that he is a ZZ homozygote.
    c Alpha-1-antitrypsin is inherited as a codominant trait with the
        locus on chromosome 14. So far 23 alleles have been identified
        of which the M allele is by far the commonest. Only the Z allele
        causes disease and then only in the homozygote. Some ZZ
        homozygotes remain asymptomatic but most develop
        emphysema in the third or fourth decades and 10% have
        neonatal liver disease.
    d His wife's alpha-1-antitrypsin status needs to be determined.
        Provided she is MM (88% of the population) all of their children
        will be unaffected MZ heterozygotes. If she is an MZ
        heterozygote (1 in 33 of the population) there would be a 1 in
        2 risk of a ZZ child. Prenatal diagnosis is possible by molecular
        analysis of fetal DNA obtained by chorionic villus sampling or
        amniocentesis.

26 Androgen insensitivity syndrome
    a Lack of pubic and body hair with normal breast development
        and female body proportions is the typical phenotype of
        complete androgen insensitivity syndrome (testicular
        feminization syndrome).
    b Testes may be palpable in the inguinal region or labia majora. If
        not, the testes are likely to be intra-abdominal.
    c Androgen insensitivity is due to deficiency of a specific cytosol
        binding protein for testosterone and dihydrotestosterone
        demonstrable in cultured genital skin fibroblasts. Normal testes
        are present and produce Müllerian inhibiting factor causing
        regression of the fetal Müllerian duct system, but
        unresponsiveness to androgens prevents induction of the
        Wolffian duct system or masculinization of the external
        genitalia. Androgen insensitivity also explains the paucity of
        pubic and body hair after puberty. Normal testes synthesize
        some oestrogen and this unopposed by androgens is
        responsible for breast development.
    d X-linked recessive.
    e All patients are infertile. Intelligence and life span are normal.
        The testes should be removed because of the risk of neoplasia
        (5−20%).

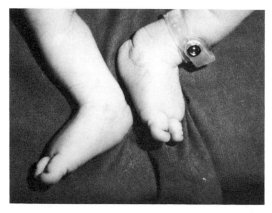

27 This is a newborn female.
   a What diagnosis should be considered?
   b How could this be confirmed?
   c What are the features of this disorder?
   d What is the recurrence risk?

28 A couple request genetic counselling because the man had a sister who died of cystic fibrosis.
   a What is the risk to their offspring?
   b Is carrier detection possible?
   c Is prenatal diagnosis possible?

27 Turner's syndrome.

  a A female neonate with lymphoedema is suggestive of Turner's syndrome.

  b Chromosome analysis. A single X chromosome (45,X) is found in most cases; 17% have an isochromosome for the long arm of the X chromosome; 16% are mosaic and 10% have a short arm deletion of one X chromosome. The Turner's syndrome phenotype is associated with deletion of the short arm, whilst long arm deletions produce streak gonads.

  c Short stature (adult height of 125–150 cm) with primary amenorrhoea and infertility (unless mosaic). Congenital heart disease, notably coarctation of the aorta and atrial septal defect, is present in 20% of cases and there is also an increased risk of unexplained hypertension (27%). Intelligence and lifespan are usually normal.

  d The overall incidence is 1 in 2500 female births and the recurrence risk is probably not higher than this.

28 a Cystic fibrosis is an autosomal recessive condition. The man's risk of being a carrier is $\frac{2}{3}$ (see footnote) and his wife has the general population carrier risk of 1 in 20. If they are both carriers 1 in 4 of their offspring will be affected. Therefore their risk of a child with cystic fibrosis is 1 in 120 ($\frac{2}{3} \times \frac{1}{20} \times \frac{1}{4}$).

  b No.

  c Prenatal diagnostic tests currently being evaluated depend on assay of microvillar enzymes (alkaline phosphatase isoenzymes and gamma-glutamyl transpeptidase) in the amniotic fluid at 18 weeks gestation and ultrasound demonstration of meconium ileus which is present in many affected fetuses. It appears that 80–90% of affected pregnancies can be detected in this way. Unfortunately the specificity of the biochemical tests is only 90–95%. This is adequate for pregnancies at 1 in 4 risk but in lower risk situations such as the present case the predictive value of a positive result becomes so low that the test cannot be recommended.

Footnote: Both the man's parents are carriers and have affected, carrier and normal offspring in the ratio 1:2:1. Since the man is not affected the first possibility is excluded so that the odds on him being a carrier rather than being normal are 2:1.

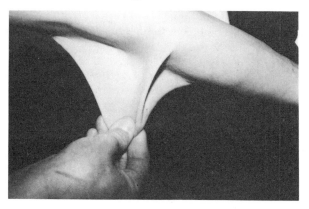

29 **a** What is the likely diagnosis?
   b What other clinical features may be found?
   c What is the mode of inheritance?
   d What is the prognosis?

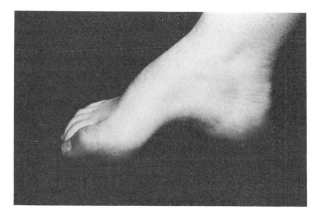

30 This 12-year-old girl complains of increasing difficulty with
   walking. She has an ataxic gait, dysarthria, an intention tremor,
   absent ankle jerks and extensor plantar responses. Her parents are
   first cousins.
   a What is the likely diagnosis?
   b What are the other clinical features of this disorder?
   c What is the prognosis?
   d What is the mode of inheritance?

29 a Ehlers–Danlos syndrome.
  b Skin hyperelasticity, poor wound healing with tissue paper scars, lax joints and easy bruising.
  c There are at least 16 distinct variants of Ehlers–Danlos syndrome (genetic heterogeneity). The commonest types are autosomal dominant but X-linked and autosomal recessive forms are known.
  d The commonest variants do not influence lifespan but in some rare types there is fragility of major blood vessels and premature death.

30 Friedreich's ataxia
  a The combination of pes cavus, progressive ataxia affecting upper and lower limbs, absent ankle jerks and extensor plantar responses is characteristic of Friedreich's ataxia.
  b Scoliosis is common. Vibration and joint position sense may be lost, especially in the feet. Cardiomyopathy and diabetes mellitus are frequent complications.
  c Disability is progressive and patients become wheelchair bound in adolescence or early adult life. The average age at death is 40 years.
  d Classic Friedreich's ataxia is autosomal recessive. Parental consanguinity is found in 5% of families, providing support for this mode of inheritance when present. Carrier detection and prenatal diagnosis are not possible. Numerous less common hereditary ataxias are known. As a generalization, those with onset in childhood or adolescence tend to be autosomal recessive whilst disorders with later onset are likely to be autosomal dominant.

31 A neonate presents with jaundice, vomiting and hepatomegaly. A urine specimen gives a positive result with Clinitest but negative with Clinistix.
  a What diagnosis must be considered?
  b What immediate management is required?
  c How could this diagnosis be confirmed?
  d What is the longterm management and prognosis?
  e What is the mode of inheritance?

32 A man presents with portal hypertension and altered behaviour. Ocular examination reveals brownish pigment at the periphery of his corneas.
  a What is the likely diagnosis?
  b How may this diagnosis be confirmed?
  c What is the risk to his children?
  d What is the prognosis?
  e What family studies are indicated?

31 **a** **Galactosaemia.**
 b Stop milk intake and correct fluid and electrolyte imbalance.
 c The urine contains the reducing substance galactose and red cell galactose-1-phosphate uridyl transferase (GALT) is absent.
 d Lifelong exclusion of milk and milk products from the diet is necessary. If this is started early enough lifespan and intelligence are usually normal, but delay beyond one month carries a high risk of mental retardation, cataracts and hepatic cirrhosis.
 e This is an autosomal recessive disorder and the recurrence risk is 1 in 4. The GALT locus is on chromosome 9. Carrier detection is possible by assay of red cell GALT. Prenatal diagnosis is also possible by assay of GALT in cultured amniotic fluid cells but it is doubtful if termination of an affected pregnancy is justified for a treatable condition.

32 **Wilson's disease**
 a Kayser–Fleischer rings are pathognomonic of Wilson's disease (hepatolenticular degeneration). They are due to deposition of copper in Descemet's membrane. Copper also accumulates in the liver causing cirrhosis, in the brain (particularly the basal ganglia) causing disturbance of motor function and behaviour, and in the renal tubules.
 b Serum caeruloplasmin is reduced and urinary copper excretion is increased. Glycosuria, proteinuria and generalized aminoaciduria may be present. Liver biopsy would show cirrhosis and increased copper content.
 c This is an autosomal recessive disorder so that all his children would be asymptomatic carriers. The risk that his wife is a carrier for this disorder is 1 in 200, so that the risk of a child with Wilson's disease is 1 in 400 (1/200 × ½).
 d D-penicillamine chelates copper and can prevent and to some extent reverse the neurological and hepatic complications.
 e This man's siblings have a 1 in 4 risk of Wilson's disease and should be screened with liver function tests and measurement of serum caeruloplasmin concentration and urinary copper excretion. If these results are normal, liver biopsy and measurement of hepatic copper content should be considered in younger sibs.

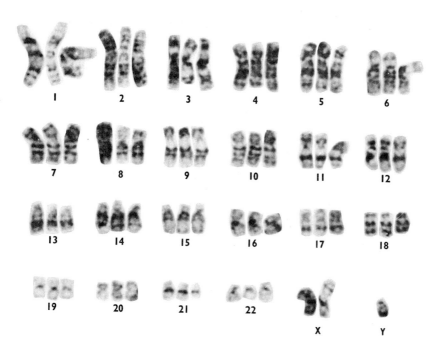

33 a What does this fetal karyotype show?
    b What would be the findings in the fetus?
    c What is the prognosis?
    d How does this abnormality arise?
    e What is the recurrence risk?

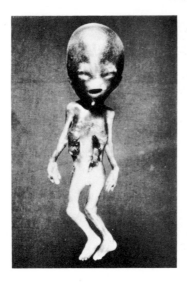 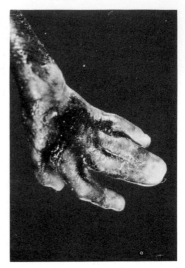

33   Triploidy

a   Triploidy with 69 chromosomes instead of the usual diploid number of 46.

b   A typical triploid fetus is extremely light for dates with a small trunk in relation to the size of the head and syndactyly as shown above. The placenta is large and may show hydatidiform change.

c   Spontaneous abortion is usual and survival to term is exceptional.

d   In most cases the extra haploid set of chromosomes is paternally derived with 66% due to double fertilization, 24% due to fertilization with a diploid sperm and 10% due to fertilization of a diploid egg. 60% are 69,XXY and most of the remainder are 69,XXX. Hydatidiform change is found only when there is a double paternal contribution.

e   Triploidy occurs in 2% of all conceptions but most abort spontaneously. The risk does not appear to be increased in subsequent pegnancies.

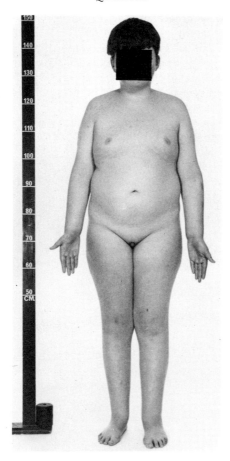

34 This 11-year-old boy is mentally retarded.

   a What abnormalities are apparent and what is the most likely
      diagnosis?
   b Why is chromosome analysis indicated?
   c What is the recurrence risk?

34 Prader–Willi syndrome

  a The central obesity, small hands and feet, small penis and
    cryptorchidism are typical of the Prader–Willi syndrome. The
    obesity develops during childhood and may be complicated by
    diabetes mellitus in adolescence. Hypogonadotrophic
    hypogonadism may be present. In infancy hypotonia is a
    prominent feature.

  b Some cases have a small deletion of the long arm of
    chromosome 15 at band q11–13 demonstrated by high
    resolution prometaphase banding.

  c This condition is usually sporadic with a low recurrence risk
    provided it is not associated with a balanced chromosome
    rearrangement in one of the parents.

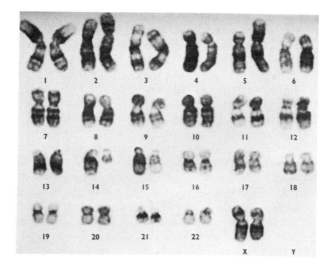

35 **This is the karyotype of the mother of a mentally retarded dysmorphic boy.**
  a What is the abnormality in this karyotype?
  b How is this related to the child's problem?
  c What is the recurrence risk?
  d What other tests are necessary?

36 **A one-week-old male infant presents with vomiting and lethargy. Biochemical analysis reveals: Plasma sodium 120 mmol/1**
                    Plasma potassium 6.8 mmol/1
  a What is the likely diagnosis?
  b How may this diagnosis be confirmed?
  c What is the prognosis?
  d What is the recurrence risk?

35 Reciprocal translocation

a There is a reciprocal translocation between chromosomes 5 and 14. This is a balanced rearrangement because the normal number of genes are still present.

b The carrier of a balanced translocation may produce offspring with chromosomal imbalance. In this case the boy inherited a normal chromosome 14 from his mother but the derivative chromosome 5. He therefore has one copy (monosomy) of the genes on the tip of the short arm of chromosome 5 and three copies (trisomy) of the genes on much of the long arm of chromosome 14.

c The risk of a handicapped child for a carrier of a reciprocal translocation depends on the mode of ascertainment. In this case ascertainment resulted from the birth of a handicapped child (rather than from investigation of recurrent miscarriages) which demonstrates that a viable pregnancy is possible despite the chromosome imbalance. Taking into account the position of the breakpoints the recurrence risk is likely to be about 10% and prenatal diagnosis should be considered in a future pregnancy.

d It is mandatory to analyse the chromosomes of other family members who might carry the balanced translocation and be at risk of having a handicapped child.

36 Congenital adrenal hyperplasia

a The combination of vomiting, hyponatraemia and hyperkalaemia should suggest congenital adrenal hyperplasia. Ninety per cent of such cases are due to adrenal 21-hydroxylase deficiency and about half of these are salt losers.

b Serum 17-hydroxyprogesterone and ACTH are both elevated. Urinary sodium and chloride are increased and pregnanetriol is raised.

c Lifelong replacement therapy with glucocorticoid is necessary. Salt-losers also need mineralocorticoid. With treatment, normal growth and intelligence are to be expected. Affected females may be born with ambiguous genitalia due to the virilizing effect of elevated levels of androgens.

d This condition is autosomal recessive with a 1 in 4 recurrence risk. 21-hydroxylase deficiency is linked to the HLA gene cluster on chromosome 6. Prenatal diagnosis can be achieved by measurement of 17-hydroxyprogesterone in amniotic fluid but it is doubtful if termination of an affected pregnancy is justified for a treatable condition.

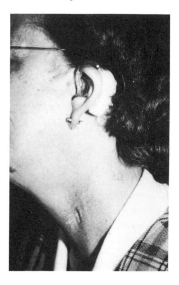

37 a What is the likely diagnosis?
    b What test is required?
    c What is the prognosis?
    d What is the mode of inheritance?

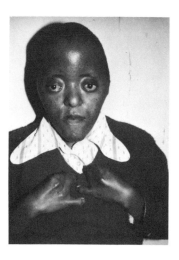

38 This girl has normal parents.
    a What abnormalities are apparent and what is the diagnosis?
    b What is the prognosis?
    c What is the recurrence risk for the parents?
    d What is the risk to the girl's offspring?

37 Branchio-oto-renal syndrome

   a The combination of deafness, cup-shaped ears, preauricular tags (note the scar in front of the ear) and branchial sinus or fistula (scar on the neck) suggests the branchio-oto-renal or BOR syndrome.

   b Renal ultrasound is indicated because there is usually renal hypoplasia or other kidney malformation.

   c Intelligence is normal and life expectancy is only reduced if renal hypoplasia is severe and results in chronic renal failure.

   d Autosomal dominant.

38 Apert syndrome

   a Syndactyly and acrocephaly due to premature closure of sutures (craniosynostosis) are the features of Apert syndrome.

   b Craniostenosis can result in brain compression and mental retardation unless relieved by linear craniectomy.

   c This is an autosomal dominant trait with full penetrance. Since the parents are normal their affected daughter must represent a new mutation and the recurrence risk would be negligible if they had more children.

   d For the girl's offspring the recurrence risk is 1 in 2. In practice most patients with this condition do not reproduce.

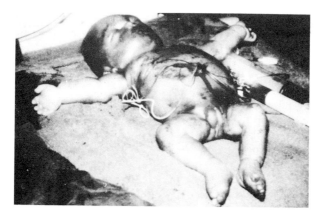

39 **This deceased newborn is Chinese.**
   a What is the likely diagnosis?
   b How may this diagnosis be confirmed?
   c What is the recurrence risk?
   d Can prenatal diagnosis be offered?

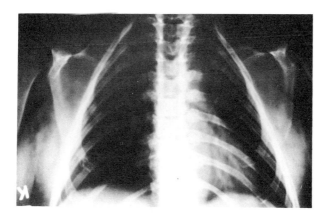

40 a What is the diagnosis?
    b What are the clinical features?
    c What is the prognosis?
    d What is the mode of inheritance?

39 Alpha thalassaemia

a Generalized oedema and neonatal death in a Chinese family suggests homozygous alpha thalassaemia.

b The child has no functioning alpha globin genes whereas normally there are two on each chromosome 16 making a total of four ($\alpha\alpha/\alpha\alpha$). There is severe anaemia and the predominant haemoglobin present has four gamma chains (Hemoglobin Barts).

c Each parent will have two alpha genes on one chromosome 16 and none on the other ($--/\alpha\alpha$). 25% of their offspring will be affected ($--/--$); 50% will be carriers like the parents ($--/\alpha\alpha$); and 25% will have normal globin genes ($\alpha\alpha/\alpha\alpha$). Screening of relatives for the carrier status is not possible on routine haematological tests.

d Molecular studies usually reveal that the alpha globin genes are missing because of a deletion of that segment of chromosome 16. DNA probes from this region will fail to identify a complementary segment in an affected fetus. This permits prenatal diagnosis using DNA obtained by chorionic villus sampling or amniocentesis.

40 Cleidocranial dysplasia

a Absence of the clavicles is a characteristic feature of cleidocranial dysplasia (cleidocranial dysostosis).

b There is short stature and defective development of the skull and clavicles. The fontanelles are large at birth and closure is delayed. If the clavicles are completely absent the shoulders can be approximated anteriorly.

c Normal lifespan and intelligence.

d Autosomal dominant.

41 A couple seek advice following the discovery of a ventricular septal defect in their first child.
   a What is the likely aetiology of this abnormality?
   b What is the recurrence risk?

42 A woman with insulin-dependent diabetes mellitus requests counselling.
   a What is the risk to her offspring of insulin-dependent diabetes mellitus?
   b What are the other risks to her offspring?

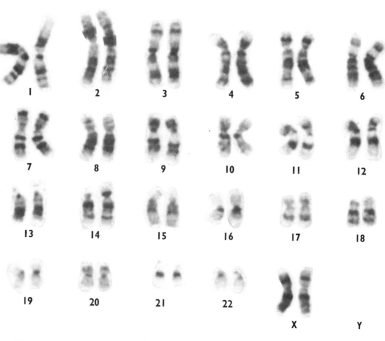

43 This is the karyotype of a baby with the clinical features of Down's syndrome.
   a What is the abnormality?
   b What is the prognosis?
   c What other tests are indicated?
   d What is the recurrence risk?

41 Congenital heart disease

  a Congenital heart disease is usually of unknown aetiology but
       shows a recurrence pattern consistent with polygenic
       inheritance. Environmental agents such as rubella are
       sometimes responsible. Chromosome aberrations, single gene
       disorders and non-Mendelian syndromes should be considered
       if other abnormalities are also present.

  b For common defects such as VSD, ASD and Fallot's tetralogy the
       recurrence risk is about 3%, and this is also the risk to the
       offspring of affected individuals. For rarer defects the risk is
       usually lower, in the range 1–2%. If two siblings are affected
       the risk to subsequent children is about 10%.

42 Diabetes Mellitus

  a Insulin-dependent diabetes mellitus is probably heterogeneous
       and this may explain the disparity in estimates of the
       recurrence risk in different studies. In most cases the risk of
       clinical diabetes in sibs or offspring is low and in the region of
       3%.

  b The incidence of major congenital malformations, notably
       congenital heart disease, spina bifida and sacral agenesis are
       increased. These complications can be minimized by skilled
       medical and obstetric management before and during the
       pregnancy.

43 Translocation Down's syndrome

  a There are three copies of chromosome 21, one of which is
       translocated to chromosome 14.

  b The phenotype is indistinguishable from the commoner type of
       Down's syndrome due to three separate copies of
       chromosome 21.

  c Chromosome analysis of both parents is mandatory. This may
       be a *de novo* rearrangement but it is more likely that one parent
       carries a balanced translocation and has one chromosome 14,
       one chromosome 21 and a third chromosome consisting of a
       14 and 21 joined together. This gives 45 chromosomes in all but
       no imbalance of genetic material since the normal number of
       genes are present and no clinical abnormality. If this is the case
       then chromosome analysis of other family members who may
       be translocation carriers and at risk of having offspring with
       Down's syndrome is also mandatory.

  d Down's syndrome will recur in 15% of the offspring if the
       mother is a balanced 14/21 translocation carrier but in only 1%
       of the offspring if the father is the carrier. Prenatal diagnosis by
       chorion villus sampling or amniocentesis can be offered.

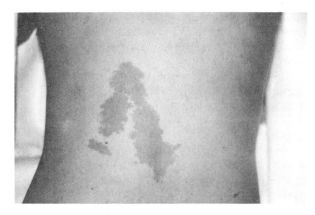

44 **This 5-year-old girl has precocious puberty.**
   a What is the diagnosis?
   b What other features may occur?
   c What is the prognosis?
   d What is the mode of inheritance?

45 **A couple contemplating marriage seek advice because they are first cousins. The man's older brother died in infancy from Pompe's disease.**
   a Is marriage between first cousins legal?
   b Are the offspring of first cousins at any increased risk?
   c What is the mode of inheritance of Pompe's disease?
   d What is the risk of this couple having a child with Pompe's disease?

44 a McCune-Albright syndrome.
   b Bony fibrous dysplasia, especially in the long bones and pelvis.
       Affected bones are prone to fracture. Hyperthyroidism or
       Cushing syndrome may develop.
   c Skull involvement may cause cranial nerve compression. Short
       stature is common. Fertility is not impaired.
   d This is a sporadic disorder.

45 Consanguinity
   a First cousin marriage is legal in the United Kingdom but illegal
       in some other countries including many states of the USA.
   b Everyone carries a small number of harmful recessive genes but
       there is a greater chance of both partners being carriers for the
       same disorder if they have grandparents in common. As a result
       the risk of an abnormal pregnancy for first cousin parents is 5%,
       double that for the general population. The risk is higher if
       there is a close family history of a serious autosomal recessive
       disorder, as in this case.
   c Pompe's disease (Glycogen storage disease type II) is an
       autosomal recessive disorder caused by deficiency of the
       lysosomal enzyme acid maltase. Massive accumulation of
       glycogen in heart muscle results in cardiac failure and death at
       around 12 months of age.

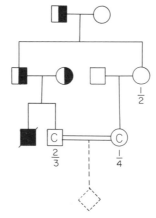

Risk of affected offspring $= \frac{1}{4} \times \frac{2}{3} \times \frac{1}{4} = \frac{1}{24}$

   d Carrier risks are given on the family pedigree above. The carrier
       risk for the man is 2/3 (see footnote). Both of his parents must
       be carriers and also one of his grandparents (shown as the
       grandfather for ease of illustration). It follows that the carrier
       risk for the woman is 1/4. Their risk of a child with Pompe's

46 A 30-year-old woman is referred with colicky abdominal pain, vomiting and upper limb weakness. Abdominal and pelvic signs are minimal. Heart rate is 140 beats/minute.
   a What metabolic disorder should be considered?
   b How would this diagnosis be confirmed?
   c What is the mode of inheritance?
   d How can the risk of further attacks be reduced?

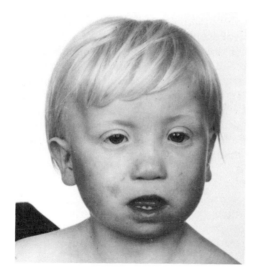

47 This child was small for gestational age at birth.
   a What is the diagnosis?
   b What other features may be found?
   c What is the recurrence risk?

continued from p. 58

disease is 1/24 as shown. Enzyme assay in leukocytes or cultured skin fibroblasts should permit their carrier status to be determined. Prenatal diagnosis is possible by assay of acid maltase in cultured amniotic fluid cells.

Footnote: Carrier parents have affected, carrier and normal offspring in the ratio 1:2:1. Since the man is not affected with Pompe's disease the first possibility can be excluded and the odds on him being a carrier rather than being normal are 2:1.

46   Acute porphyria

   a   Acute porphyria should be considered. Acute intermittent
         porphyria is the commonest type but variegate porphyria and
         hereditary coproporphyria can present in the same way.
         Photo-sensitivity is a common feature of variegate porphyria.

   b   During attacks the urine contains large amounts of the
         porphyrin precursors 5-aminolaevulinic acid (ALA) and
         porphobilinogen (PBG). The excretion pattern of porphyrins in
         urine and faeces allows the three types to be distinguished.
         Red cell porphobilinogen deaminase is reduced in acute
         intermittent porphyria.

   c   Autosomal dominant. Other family members at risk should be
         screened and counselled. About 50% of gene carriers show
         abnormal urinary and faecal excretion of porphyrins and
         precursors. If no abnormality is found specific enzyme assay
         should be undertaken.

   d   Restrict alcohol intake and avoid drugs which may precipitate
         an acute attack, for example barbiturates, sulphonamides,
         phenytoin and oral contraceptives. Check before prescribing
         any drug.

47   Fetal alcohol syndrome

   a   The short palpebral fissures, small nose and smooth philtrum
         are suggestive of the fetal alcohol syndrome.

   b   Mental retardation (usually mild), moderate microcephaly and
         congenital heart disease.

   c   There is a high risk of recurrence if the mother is unable to
         moderate her alcohol intake.

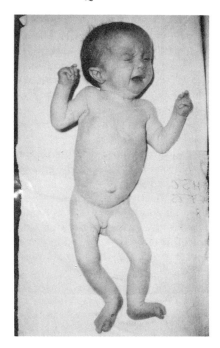

48 This newborn is small for gestational age.
   a What is the likely diagnosis?
   b How could this diagnosis be confirmed?
   c What is the prognosis?
   d What is the recurrence risk?

49 A couple request counselling because the woman's father has haemophilia B (Christmas disease).
   a What is the risk to their offspring?
   b Is carrier detection possible?
   c Is prenatal diagnosis possible?

48   Trisomy 18

a   Clenched hands with overlapping index and fifth fingers,
    prominent occiput, small chin, low-set malformed ears, short
    big toes and rocker bottom feet in a small for gestational age
    neonate suggest trisomy 18. Other common features are a short
    sternum, cryptorchidism in males and a dermal ridge pattern of
    eight or more arches.

b   Chromosome analysis to confirm the presence of an additional
    chromosome 18.

c   These infants show profound developmental delay. Multiple
    congenital malformations are usually present and only 10%
    survive beyond the first year of life.

d   The incidence of trisomy 18 is 1 in 3000 live births. The
    recurrence risk in young mothers is not established but by
    analogy with trisomy 21 may be as high as 1.5%. In women
    over 35 years of age this is exceeded by the increasing risk of
    chromosome abnormalities in older mothers.

49   Haemophilia B

a   She is an obligate carrier for this X-linked recessive disorder.
    Thus on average half of her sons will be affected and half of her
    daughters will be carriers.

b   Carrier detection is possible by a combination of
    haematological tests and DNA analysis.

c   Prenatal diagnosis formerly required fetal blood sampling for
    factor IX assay in male pregnancies. In many families earlier
    prenatal diagnosis is now possible by DNA analysis after
    chorionic villus sampling.

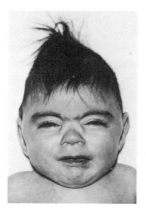

50 a What is the diagnosis?
    b What other features may occur?
    c What is the prognosis?
    d What is the recurrence risk?

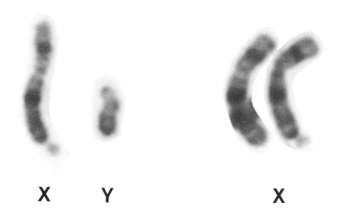

X   Y   X

51 This is a partial karyotype showing the sex chromosomes from a
    mentally retarded male. His mother's sex chromosomes are also
    shown.
    a What is the diagnosis?
    b What other clinical features may be present?
    c How is this condition inherited?
    d What further investigations are required?

50   de Lange syndrome

    a Synophrys (eyebrows joining across the midline) with a depressed nasal bridge, small nose, anteverted nostrils, thin upper lip and downturning mouth are characteristic of de Lange syndrome.

    b Very short stature, microcephaly, severe mental retardation, limb defects and congenital heart disease.

    c Death in early childhood is usual.

    d A chromosome abnormality should be excluded. In most cases the aetiology is unknown and the empiric recurrence risk is 1 in 50.

51   Fragile X syndrome

    a There is a secondary constriction or fragile site near the tip of the long arm of the X chromosome. This abnormality is associated with mental retardation and is called the fragile X syndrome. The mother is a carrier since one of her X chromosomes shows the fragile site.

    b Enlarged testes, especially after puberty, elongated facies and large ears. The mental retardation varies from mild to severe with a tendency to repetitive speech.

    c This is an X-linked recessive trait with mild mental retardation in 20–30% of the female carriers.

    d Female relatives should be screened to identify carriers by karyotyping in culture medium deficient in thymidine and folic acid. Unfortunately cytogenetic detection of the fragile X is only possible in about 50% of the female carriers with normal intelligence.

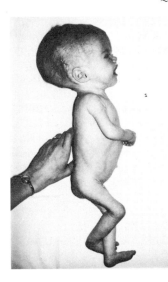 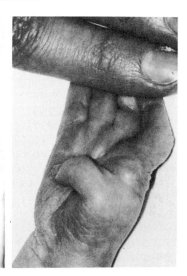

52 **This boy's brother had the same condition.**
   a What does this show and what is the likely diagnosis?
   b What is the prognosis?
   c What is the recurrence risk?
   d Is prenatal diagnosis possible?

53 **A mentally retarded boy is found to have a positive urinary cyanide-nitroprusside test.**
   a What is the probable diagnosis?
   b What other physical features may be present?
   c How could this diagnosis be confirmed?
   d What is the prognosis for this condition?
   e What is the recurrence risk?

52 X-linked hydrocephalus
  a This child has hydrocephalus and hypoplastic flexed thumbs. The thumbs are a diagnostic clue that this is the rare X-linked recessive type of hydrocephalus due to aqueduct stenosis.
  b The prognosis is poor. Despite shunting, mental retardation is the rule.
  c The mother is an obligate carrier as she has had two affected sons. On average half of her sons will be affected and half of her daughters will be carriers. Female relatives on the maternal side may also be carriers and should be offered genetic counselling.
  d Prenatal diagnosis prior to the third trimester may be possible by serial ultrasound measurements of the ventricle to mantle ratio.

53 a Homocystinuria.
  b Dislocated lenses, marfanoid habitus, stiff joints and a malar flush.
  c The diagnosis is supported by elevated levels of homocystine and methionine in the blood and persistent urinary excretion of homocystine. Cystathionine synthase is markedly reduced in cultured skin fibroblasts in the commonest form of this disease.
  d Untreated, two-thirds of patients develop mental retardation and life expectancy is reduced because of thromboembolic episodes. Diagnosis by newborn screening and early treatment with pyridoxine (vitamin B6) in some cases and/or dietary restriction of methionine permits normal intellectual development.
  e This is an autosomal recessive trait with a 1 in 4 recurrence risk. Prenatal diagnosis is possible by enzyme assay in cultured amniotic fluid cells.

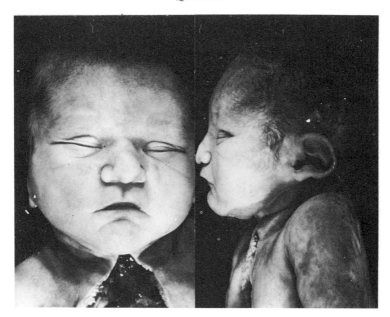

54 **This baby did not establish adequate spontaneous respiration after birth.**

   a What does the picture show?

   b What is the most likely diagnosis?

   c What is the prognosis?

   d What is the recurrence risk?

   e Is prenatal diagnosis available?

54 Potter syndrome

  a The large low-set ears and squashed facies are typical of Potter
     syndrome. Other features include dry wrinkled skin, spade-like
     hands, genital anomalies and pulmonary hypoplasia.

  b This syndrome can be secondary to oligohydramnios of any
     cause but is most commonly associated with renal tract
     abnormalities, particularly bilateral renal agenesis.

  c Pulmonary hypoplasia usually results in early neonatal death.

  d The empiric recurrence risk for bilateral renal agenesis is
     1 in 33. There is an increased frequency of renal anomalies
     (hypoplasia and unilateral agenesis) detected by ultrasound in
     the parents of such children but it is unclear how this affects the
     recurrence risk.

  e Prenatal diagnosis is possible by ultrasound to detect
     oligohydramnios and demonstrate absent kidneys with failure
     of the bladder to fill and empty.

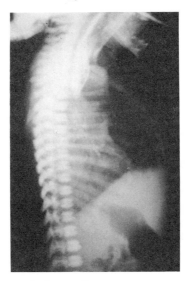

55 **This infant has a missing radius.**
   a What is the probable diagnosis?
   b What is the prognosis?
   c What is the recurrence risk?

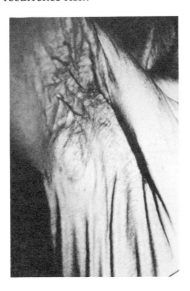

56 **a** What is the diagnosis?
   b What is the characteristic ocular finding?
   c What are the complications?
   d What is the mode of inheritance?

55   VATER association.
   a The combination of radial limb defects and oesophageal atresia
         suggests the VATER association. The components of this
         association are *V*ertebral defects, *A*nal atresia,
         *T*racheo-*E*sophageal fistula and oesophageal atresia, *R*adial
         and *R*enal defects, and congenital heart disease.
   b Intelligence is normal and the prognosis depends on the extent
         to which the malformations are surgically correctable.
   c This is a sporadic condition with a low recurrence risk.

56   Pseudoxanthoma elasticum
   a The skin is yellowish and thickened with a cobbled and ridged
         surface and forms lax folds. Body folds are typically affected,
         particularly the neck and axilla.
   b Angioid streaks in the retina.
   c Coronary and peripheral vascular insufficiency and
         gastrointestinal haemorrhage are common and result from
         degeneration of arterial elastic fibres. Vascular insufficiency can
         also cause a variety of neurological signs and symptoms.
         Hypertension is common and probably due to renal vascular
         disease. Vision may be impaired by fundal haemorrhage.
   d There are autosomal dominant and autosomal recessive forms.
         These are clinically indistinguishable so that counselling of an
         isolated case is difficult.

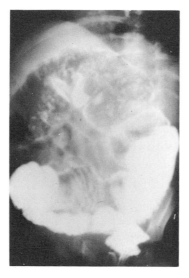

57 a What is the likely diagnosis?
    b How may this diagnosis be confirmed?
    c What is the recurrence risk?
    d Is prenatal diagnosis available?

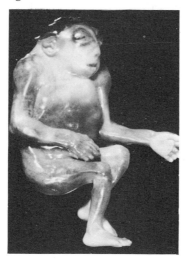

58 a What is the diagnosis?
    b What is the prognosis?
    c What is the recurrence risk?
    d How might the risk of recurrence be reduced?
    e Is prenatal diagnosis available?

57 a Hirschsprung disease (colonic aganglionosis).
   b Rectal biopsy confirms the absence of submucosal and
      myenteric ganglion cells.
   c Hirschsprung disease is inherited as a multifactorial trait. It is
      much commoner in males than females and so the recurrence
      risk depends on the sex of the index case. If a male child is
      affected the empiric risk is 1 in 25 whereas for a female index
      case the recurrence risk is 1 in 8. The risk is increased if the
      aganglionic segment is long and decreased if only a short
      segment of the bowel is involved.
   d No.

58 a Anencephaly.
   b Neonatal death is invariable.
   c In subsequent pregnancies there is an increased risk of neural
      tube defects (anencephaly and spina bifida) which is
      approximately ten times the local population incidence. In the
      West of Scotland the incidence is 4 per 1000 and the recurrence
      risk about 4%. After two affected pregnancies the recurrence
      risk is at least 10%.
   d There is evidence to suggest that vitamin supplementation
      started at least one month before conception and continued past
      the time when the neural tube closes (4 weeks from conception)
      reduces the recurrence risk. Folic acid alone may be effective
      but the most widely used preparation (Pregnavite Forte F,
      Bencard) also contains other vitamins which could be
      important. Research is in progress to clarify this issue.
   e For pregnancies at high risk because of a previous neural tube
      defect, prenatal diagnosis by ultrasound scanning and
      amniocentesis for amniotic fluid alphafetoprotein assay is
      recommended.

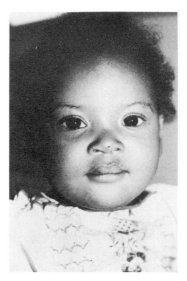

59 **This girl has the karyotype 47, XXX.**
   a What are the clinical features of this chromosome abnormality?
   b What is the recurrence risk in subsequent children?
   c What would be the risk of chromosome abnormalities in this girl's offspring?

60 **A 50-year-old man presents with lethargy and massive splenomegaly. His blood shows: Hb 10.6 g/dl, WCC 370 × 10⁹/l with a differential count of neutrophils 47%, myelocytes 10%, metamyelocytes 6%, promyelocytes 19%, basophils 7%, eosinophils 6%, lymphocytes 2% and blasts 3%.**
   a What is the likely diagnosis?
   b What is the associated chromosome abnormality?
   c How may this be related to the disease?
   d What is the recurrence risk?

59 Triple X

  a Girls with triple X do not have any characteristic physical features and the majority are never diagnosed. Intelligence quotients are shifted to the left and 15% have an IQ below 70.

  b The incidence of triple X increases with advancing maternal age but remains small compared to the risk for trisomy 21. It is not known whether the risk is increased after an affected pregnancy.

  c Most affected individuals are fertile but there may be an association with premature ovarian failure. An increased frequency of 47, XXX and 47, XXY offspring might be expected but has rarely been reported.

60 a Chronic myeloid leukæmia

  b The Philadelphia chromosome results from a reciprocal 9−22 translocation. This is found in the malignant marrow in 95% of cases.

  c The *c-abl* oncogene is translocated from its normal site at the end of the long arm of chromosome 9 to a site on 22 next to the lambda immunoglobulin light chain gene cluster. In this location the oncogene shows enhanced expression but it is not known how this relates to the development of the disease.

  d The condition is sporadic with a low recurrence risk. The translocation is not found in other family members, nor is it present whilst the patient is in remission.

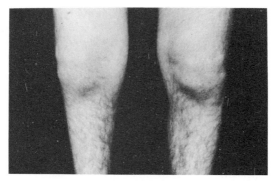

61 **This 20-year-old man has a father with the same disorder.**
  a What is the likely diagnosis?
  b What are the other features?
  c What is the prognosis?
  d What is the mode of inheritance?

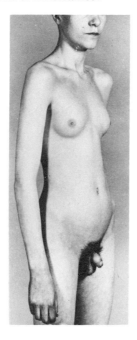

62 **This man is infertile.**
  a What is the likely diagnosis?
  b How may this be confirmed?
  c What are the clinical features of this disorder?
  d What is the recurrence risk?

61   Hereditary motor and sensory neuropathy type I
  a   Familial wasting of distal muscles (inverted champagne bottle
      legs) suggests hereditary motor and sensory neuropathy type I
      (peroneal muscular atrophy, Charcot-Marie-Tooth disease).
  b   Onset is in the teens with foot drop, absent ankle jerks,
      enlarged peripheral nerves and some sensory loss especially for
      vibration. Nerve conduction velocities are reduced.
  c   Lifespan is normal with mild to moderate disability.
  d   Usually autosomal dominant.

62   Klinefelter's syndrome
  a   Infertility and gynaecomastia suggest Klinefelter's syndrome.
  b   Chromosome analysis shows 47, XXY
  c   Infertility due to azoospermia is a constant feature. At puberty
      the testes do not increase in size but remain small and soft.
      Gynaecomastia develops in a minority of cases. Some
      individuals have long limbs and a gynaecoid appearance but
      many do not. In the majority of cases intelligence is within the
      normal range but the IQ distribution is skewed to the left
      resulting in a substantially increased risk of mild mental
      retardation. Children with 47, XXY often show delayed
      language development and an increased frequency of behaviour
      problems at school.
  d   The incidence of 47, XXY increases with advancing maternal age
      but remains small compared to the risk for trisomy 21. It is not
      known if the risk is increased after an affected pregnancy.

63 A healthy Cypriot woman has a routine blood count at the 16th week of her first pregnancy. It reveals: Hb 11.8 g/dl; red cell count 5.83 × 10⁹/l; MCV 62fl and MCH 20.5 pg.

   a What is the likely diagnosis?
   b How may this diagnosis be confirmed?
   c What action is necessary?

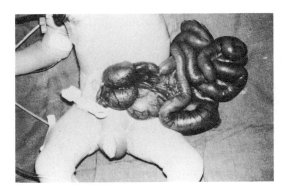

64   **a** What is the diagnosis?
     b What is the prognosis?
     c What is the recurrence risk?
     d Is prenatal diagnosis available?

63 Beta thalassaemia

  a Hypochromic microcytic anaemia is commonly due to iron deficiency anaemia but in patients of Mediterranean origin beta thalassaemia trait should be suspected.

  b Haemoglobin electrophoresis in beta thalassaemia heterozygotes reveals increased amounts of haemoglobin F and haemoglobin A_2.

  c Her husband must be screened for beta thalassaemia trait because if he is also a carrier there is a 1 in 4 risk of a homozygous fetus with beta thalassaemia. In this situation prenatal diagnosis will require fetal blood sampling at 19 weeks gestation. In a future pregnancy earlier diagnosis may be possible by DNA analysis after chorionic villus sampling.

64 Gastroschisis

  a Gastroschisis: an anterior abdominal wall defect not involving the umbilical cord and without a sac.

  b Surgical correction may be difficult as multiple areas of atretic intestine commonly occur. Congenital heart disease coexists in 20%.

  c This is a sporadic malformation with a low recurrence risk.

  d Prenatal diagnosis is possible by ultrasound. These lesions cause elevated maternal serum alphafetoprotein and will usually be detected by screening programmes for neural tube defects.

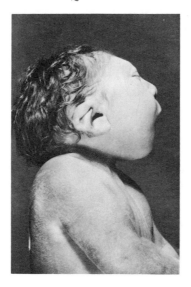

65 **The parents of this child are first cousins.**
   a What is the diagnosis?
   b What is the differential diagnosis?
   c What is the recurrence risk?
   d Is prenatal diagnosis possible?

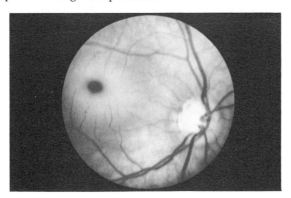

66 **This is the fundus of a 2-year-old boy from an Ashkenazi Jewish family.**
   a What is the diagnosis?
   b What are the clinical features of this disorder?
   c What is the recurrence risk?
   d Is carrier detection possible?
   e Is prenatal diagnosis possible?

65 a Microcephaly.
   b Craniosynostosis needs to be excluded. Primary microcephaly is
        due to failure of brain growth which can result from congenital
        infection, birth trauma, a chromosome abnormality or maternal
        phenylketonuria. In all of these cases the head is small but
        usually has a normal shape. This child has the rare autosomal
        recessive type of microcephaly with a characteristic sweptback
        forehead.
   c For autosomal recessive microcephaly the recurrence risk is
        1 in 4.
   d Prenatal diagnosis may be possible with detailed ultrasound
        scanning but microcephaly is not necessarily present before the
        legal limit for termination of pregnancy.

66 a Tay-Sachs disease.
   b Infantile onset with progressive loss of previously acquired
        skills, hyperacusis, spasticity, seizures and a cherry-red spot on
        the macula lutea. Most affected children are dead by 4 years of
        age.
   c This is an autosomal recessive disorder with a 1 in 4 recurrence
        risk. The carrier frequency in Ashkenazi Jews is particularly
        high, about 1 in 30, giving a birth incidence in this ethnic
        group of 1 in 3600 ($1/30 \times 1/30 \times 1/4$).
   d Tay-Sachs disease is due to deficiency of the lysosomal enzyme
        hexosaminidase A. Carrier detection is possible by assay of
        serum hexosaminidase and screening should be offered to other
        family members and their spouses to identify couples who are
        both carriers and at risk of having affected offspring.
        Unfortunately the test is unreliable in pregnant women.
   e Prenatal diagnosis is possible by assay of hexosaminidase A in
        cultured amniotic cells or chorionic villi.

67 A 3-month-old female infant was floppy at birth and has
    subsequently developed severe hypotonia and weakness. She is
    alert and visually responsive but shows a paucity of movement.
    There is indrawing of the chest on inspiration. Tendon jerks are
    absent and there is fasciculation of the tongue. She is the first
    child of healthy unrelated parents.
    a What is the most likely diagnosis?
    b How would this diagnosis be confirmed?
    c What is the prognosis?
    d What is the recurrence risk?

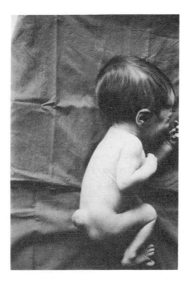

68 a What is the diagnosis?
    b Could such a lesion be detected in pregnancy by measurement
       of maternal serum alphafetoprotein?
    c What is the recurrence risk?
    d Should prenatal diagnosis be offered in a future pregnancy?

67 a Infantile spinal muscular atrophy (Werdnig-Hoffmann disease).
  b Electromyography shows denervation and muscle biopsy confirms neurogenic atrophy. The serum creatine phosphokinase is normal.
  c Death in 1–2 years from respiratory failure and food aspiration.
  d This is an autosomal recessive disorder with a 1 in 4 recurrence risk. Neither prenatal diagnosis nor carrier detection are available. Artificial insemination with donor semen (AID) or adoption are possible options.

68 Spina bifida
  a This infant has a closed neural tube defect complicated by hydrocephalus.
  b In the case of anencephaly and open spina bifida, leakage of alphafetoprotein (AFP) causes raised levels in amniotic fluid and maternal serum. However, if the neural tube defect is covered by skin (closed spina bifida) there is no leakage of AFP and these lesions cannot be identified by maternal serum screening programmes. Closed spina bifida can often be detected by careful ultrasound scanning.
  c In subsequent pregnancies there is an increased risk of neural tube defects (anencephaly and open or closed spina bifida) which is approximately ten times the local population incidence. Periconceptional vitamin supplementation may reduce the recurrence risk. (see question 58).
  d For pregnancies at high risk because of a previous neural tube defect, prenatal diagnosis by ultrasound scanning and amniocentesis for amniotic fluid alphafetoprotein assay is recommended.

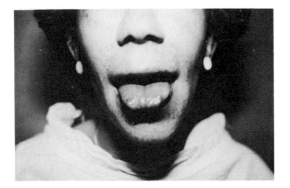

69   a   What is the diagnosis?
      b   What is the prognosis?
      c   What is the mode of inheritance?

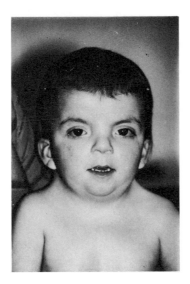

70   **This child has pulmonary stenosis and short stature with a 46,XX karyotype.**
      a   What is the likely diagnosis?
      b   What other features may be found?
      c   What is the recurrence risk?

69   Multiple endocrine neoplasia type III
   a Multiple neuromata on the tongue are pathognomonic of type
      III multiple endocrine neoplasia and are present from early
      childhood. These patients also have long thin faces and
      blubbery lips.
   b Most patients develop medullary thyroid carcinoma with
      elevated levels of serum calcitonin. Prophylactic total
      thyroidectomy should therefore be considered.
      Phaeochromocytomas may also occur.
   c Autosomal dominant.

70   Noonan syndrome
   a Short webbed neck, widely spaced eyes (hypertelorism),
      pulmonary stenosis and short stature are typical of Noonan
      syndrome. Chromosome analysis excludes 45, X Turner's
      syndrome.
   b The phenotype is variable and alters with age. Other features
      include mild to moderate mental retardation, ptosis,
      down-slanting palpebral fissures, cubitus valgus, urinary tract
      malformations and hypogonadism. Various cardiac lesions can
      occur but usually involve the right side of the heart.
   c Autosomal dominant inheritance is likely in some families. For
      normal parents the risk of recurrence in subsequent children is
      low.

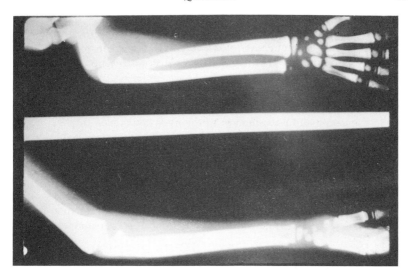

71 **a** What is the diagnosis?
    b What are the clinical features?
    c What is the mode of inheritance?

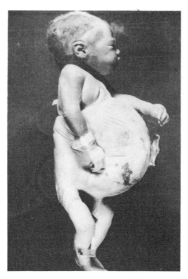

72 **a** What is the name of this condition?
    b What is the cause?
    c What is the prognosis?
    d What is the recurrence risk?

71 Osteopetrosis
   a The increased bone density is typical of osteopetrosis.
   b This condition occurs in two forms. In the severe childhood
      type the bones are brittle and prone to fracture. Bony
      overgrowth can cause cranial nerve compression with loss of
      visual acuity, extraocular muscle paralysis, facial weakness or
      nerve deafness. Obliteration of the bone marrow leads to
      anaemia and enlargement of the liver and spleen due to
      extramedullary haemopoeisis. In the adult type of osteopetrosis
      there may be a tendency to fractures but often the disorder is
      asymptomatic and discovered as an incidental radiological
      finding.
   c The adult form is autosomal dominant whereas the severe
      childhood form is autosomal recessive. Marrow transplantation
      is effective treatment for the childhood type of osteopetrosis.

72 a Prune belly syndrome.
   b Fetal obstructive uropathy results in abdominal distension and
      poor development of abdominal wall musculature.
   c The prognosis depends on the severity of the underlying renal
      lesion.
   d The recurrence risk is usually low.

73   A couple have had three first-trimester miscarriages.
  a   What proportion of pregnancies miscarry in the first trimester?
  b   What are the commonest causes of early miscarriage?
  c   What genetic tests should be offered to this couple?
  d   Do they require prenatal diagnosis in their next pregnancy?

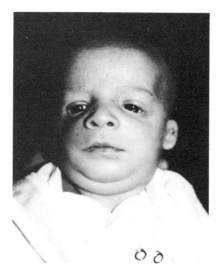

74   a   What is the diagnosis?
  b   What other clinical problems may occur?
  c   What is the mode of inheritance?

73   Recurrent miscarriages

a   15% of recognized pregnancies miscarry during the first
    trimester. The proportion is higher in older mothers.

b   60% of early spontaneous abortions are chromosomally
    abnormal (autosomal trisomy especially trisomy 16 in 30%; 45,X
    in 10%; triploidy in 10%; tetraploidy in 5%; others 5%). Ten
    per cent of early spontaneous abortions are malformed.

c   Chromosome analysis of husband and wife is indicated after
    three early miscarriages and in about 5% of cases one of them
    will be found to have a balanced chromosome rearrangement,
    for example a translocation or an inversion. This gives rise to
    conceptions with an unbalanced chromosome constitution
    which miscarry.

d   Prenatal diagnosis is not indicated in their next pregnancy
    provided they both have normal karyotypes and there is no
    other indication such as advanced maternal age.

74   Treacher Collins syndrome

a   This child has Treacher Collins syndrome (mandibulofacial
    dysostosis) with malar and mandibular hypoplasia,
    downslanting palpebral fissures and malformed ears.

b   Conductive deafness and cleft palate. There may be an
    increased risk of mental retardation.

c   This is an autosomal dominant disorder with very variable
    expression. Sixty per cent of cases are new mutations but before
    concluding that this has occurred it is essential to carefully
    examine the parents of an affected individual because mild
    micrognathia, minor ear deformity or partial absence of the
    eyelashes on the lower eyelid may be the only manifestation of
    the disorder.

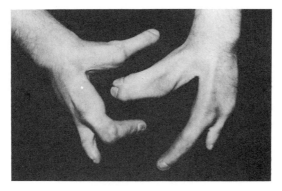

75 a What is this abnormality?
   b What is the recurrence risk?

76 A 30-year-old man requests counselling because his mother had bilateral retinoblastomas.
   a What is his risk of retinoblastoma?
   b What is the risk to his children?
   c Would the risks be the same if the retinoblastoma had been unilateral in his mother?
   d What is the connection with chromosome 13?

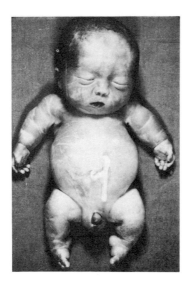

77 a What is the diagnosis?
   b What is the recurrence risk?
   c Is prenatal diagnosis available?

75 **Split-hand deformity**
a A cleft divides the hand into two parts which can move towards each other like the claws of a lobster. There is usually syndactyly between the remaining digits. Function can be surprisingly good. This defect is often called ectrodactyly but this term is also used by some authors to describe terminal transverse defects where one or more fingers are missing from an otherwise normal hand. Split-hand deformity is frequently associated with split foot.
b Many, but not all, families show autosomal dominant inheritance. Sporadic cases are often due to new dominant mutations in which case the risk to subsequent children is small but there is a substantial risk to the offspring of the affected individual.
   Typical split-hand deformity is occasionally seen as part of the EEC (ectrodactyly-ectodermal dysplasia-cleft lip/palate) syndrome which is autosomal dominant.

76 **Retinoblastoma**
a Bilateral retinoblastoma is inherited as an autosomal dominant trait but tumours only develop in childhood.
b Penetrance is incomplete and the chance that he has inherited the retinoblastoma gene but not manifested the condition is 1 in 6. The chance of his children inheriting the gene is half of this risk or 1 in 12. With a penetrance of 80% their risk of developing a retinoblastoma is 1 in 15 (80% × 1/12). They should be regularly screened by an ophthalmologist until they reach adolescence.
c Only 15% of unilateral retinoblastomas are inherited so the risks would be much lower.
d Occasionally deletion of band 13q14 is associated with retinoblastoma and this was the first clue to the site of this disease locus.

77 **Lethal short-limbed dwarfism**
a This neonate has lethal short-limbed dwarfism. Many different disorders can produce this phenotype and radiographs are essential to distinguish between them.
b Some of these conditions are autosomal recessive with a 1 in 4 recurrence risk whilst others are sporadic with a negligible risk to subsequent pregnancies: hence the importance of a precise diagnosis.
c In most cases, prenatal diagnosis is possible by serial ultrasonic measurements of limb lengths.

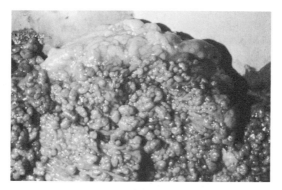

78 This is a portion of excised large bowel from a woman who died of metastatic carcinoma of the colon. The small bowel was normal.

   a What is the diagnosis?

   b What is the risk to her teenage daughter?

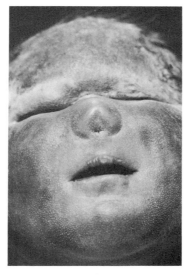

79 a What is the likely diagnosis? ·

   b What other features may occur?

   c What is the prognosis?

   d What is the recurrence risk?

78 Familial polyposis coli

a There are numerous adenomatous polyps characteristic of familial polyposis coli. Polyps are confined to the colon in this disorder.

b This is an autosomal dominant condition and the daughter has a 50% risk of inheriting the mutant gene. She should be regularly screened by endoscopy for evidence of the disorder. Polyps usually develop in adolescence and are present in the majority of gene carriers by 20 years of age. If polyps are found, total colectomy with ileostomy or subtotal colectomy with ileorectal anastomosis should be considered since malignant change is almost invariable sooner or later. If the rectum is retained it should be inspected regularly and kept free of polyps.

Polyposis of the large bowel associated with osteomas of the facial bones, epidermal or sebaceous cysts and dermoids or fibromas of the skin, particularly at the site of scars, constitutes Gardner syndrome, a distinct autosomal dominant disorder in which the risk of colonic malignancy is also high.

79 Holoprosencephaly

a Closely spaced eyes (hypotelorism) and a single central nostril reflect underlying holoprosencephaly.

b Holoprosencephaly includes variable degrees of failure of development of the forebrain and mid-face. In more severe cases there is bilateral cleft lip with absent philtrum, absent nose and a single central eye.

c This cerebral malformation usually results in death in infancy.

d Half of the cases are due to trisomy 13; otherwise the empiric recurrence risk is 6%.

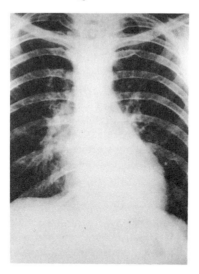

80 a What does this X-ray show?
  b What is the mode of inheritance?
  c What is the recurrence risk?

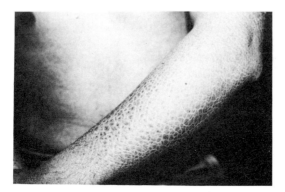

81 **This man's maternal uncle has the same skin condition.**
  a What is the likely diagnosis?
  b How could this diagnosis be confirmed?
  c What are the obstetric complications of this condition?

82 **A woman with treated phenylketonuria requests counselling.**
  a What is the recurrence risk for her offspring?
  b What else should she be told?
  c Is prenatal diagnosis possible?

80 Coarctation of the aorta
  a Rib notching due to coarctation of the aorta.
  b Isolated coarctation is usually a polygenic disorder. In a girl Turner's syndrome should be excluded.
  c The empiric recurrence risk for sibs or offspring is 1 in 50 as compared with the incidence in the general population of 1 in 1600.

81 a X-linked ichthyosis.
  b Deficiency of the enzyme steroid sulphatase can be demonstrated in hair roots, leucocytes or cultured skin fibroblasts.
  c The same disorder is known to obstetricians as placental sulphatase deficiency and manifests when a woman who is a carrier for the condition has an affected male fetus. This enzyme is an essential step in the metabolic pathway to oestriol and monitoring of urinary oestriols will give very low levels and may cause undue alarm. Furthermore, during labour inadequate cervical dilatation often necessitates operative delivery.

82 Phenylketonuria
  a Phenylketonuria is an autosomal recessive disorder so that she must be homozygous for the defective gene. All her offspring will be carriers (heterozygous) but they are only at risk of phenylketonuria if her spouse happens by chance to be a carrier for this disorder. The carrier frequency is 1 in 50 and the risk of an affected child therefore 1 in 100 ($1/2 \times 1/50$).
  b It is essential to restart a phenylalanine-restricted diet before conception and strictly monitor blood phenylalanine levels during pregnancy. Phenylalanine is concentrated on the fetal side of the placenta and elevated levels in the fetus can cause microcephaly and mental retardation.
  c The locus for phenylalanine hydroxylase is on chromosome 12 and the gene has been cloned. Prenatal diagnosis would be possible using molecular genetic techniques but it is doubtful if termination of an affected pregnancy would be justified for a treatable disorder.

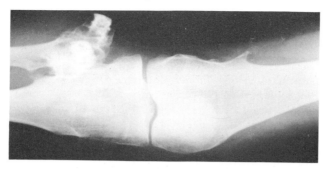

83 a What is the diagnosis?
    b What are the clinical features of this disorder?
    c What are the complications?
    d What is the mode of inheritance?

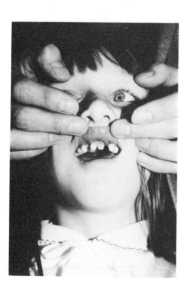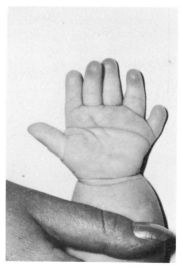

84 **This girl has short-limbed dwarfism. The photograph of her hand
    was taken in infancy.**
    a What is the likely diagnosis?
    b What other clinical features may be present?
    c What is the prognosis for height?
    d What is the mode of inheritance?
    e Is prenatal diagnosis possible?

83 Multiple exostoses

   a Exostoses are seen arising from the femur, tibia and fibula characteristic of multiple exostoses (diaphyseal aclasis).

   b Exostoses appear in childhood at sites of growing bone, particularly the long bones, scapulae, ribs and pelvis. Proliferation ceases in adolescence.

   c Exostoses can cause deformity, interfere with joint movement and compress soft tissues such as tendons and nerves. There may be shortening of involved bones. The risk of malignant change is 2%.

   d Autosomal dominant with 40% of cases due to new mutations.

84 Ellis–van Creveld syndrome

   a Short-limbed dwarfism, post-axial polydactyly and frenulae between the alveolar ridge and upper lip are typical of Ellis–van Creveld syndrome (chondroectodermal dysplasia).

   b Hypoplastic nails, defective dentition, small chest, genu valgum and congenital heart disease, especially atrial septal defect.

   c Adult height in the range 108–160 cm.

   d Autosomal recessive.

   e Prenatal diagnosis is possible by demonstrating polydactyly and shortened limbs on ultrasound scanning.

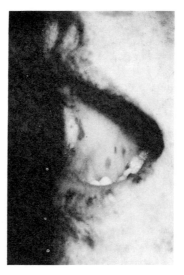

85   a   What is the diagnosis?
     b   What are the other features of this condition?
     c   What are the complications?
     d   What is the mode of inheritance?

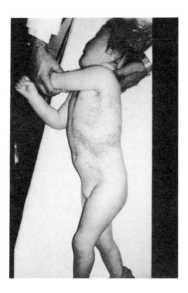

86   a   What is the diagnosis?
     b   What other features may be present?
     c   What is the mode of inheritance?

85 Peutz—Jeghers syndrome
a The circumoral and buccal pigmentation is characteristic of the Peutz—Jeghers syndrome.
b Polyposis involving the small intestine and occasionally the stomach or large bowel.
c Intestinal polyps may cause intussusception. Ovarian granulosa cell tumour occurs in 10—15% of females. The risk of intestinal malignancy is small.
d Usually autosomal dominant.

86 Incontinentia pigmenti
a The whorled pattern of pigmentation is characteristic of incontinentia pigmenti.
b Partial alopecia, hypodontia, mental retardation and ocular anomalies.
c Incontinentia pigmenti is believed to be an X-linked dominant disorder with *in utero* lethality for hemizygous males providing an explanation for the striking excess of affected females. If the mother of the child is not affected the risk of recurrence in future offspring is very small. The child's female offspring will have a 1 in 2 risk and she will also have an excess of miscarriages representing the loss of affected males.

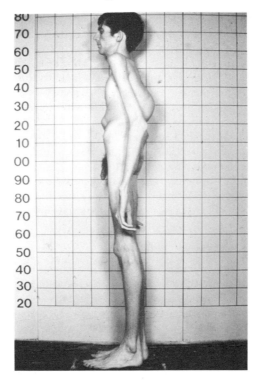

87 a What is the diagnosis?
   b What other features may be present?
   c What is the prognosis?
   d What is the mode of inheritance?

88 **A 53 year-old woman requests counselling because her father died of Huntington's chorea. Her son has just married and is also seeking advice.**
   a What is her risk of developing the disease?
   b What are the risks to her son and any children he may have?
   c What is the prognosis for someone who develops the disease?
   d Is prenatal diagnosis possible?

87   Marfan syndrome

a Long limbs resulting in altered body proportions (reduced upper to lower segment ratio), kyphoscoliosis and arachnodactyly are the typical features of the Marfan syndrome.

b Lax joints, skin striae, lens subluxation with iridodonesis, mitral valve prolapse and aortic aneurysm.

c The average lifespan is 40–50 years with aortic rupture as the commonest cause of death. Regular assessment is therefore important with measurement of the aortic root dimensions by ultrasound and aortic arch replacement in patients with evidence of progressive dilatation.

d Autosomal dominant with variable expression which may render counselling difficult in mildly affected individuals. About 15% of cases represent new mutations. Prenatal diagnosis is not possible.

88   Huntington's chorea

a Huntington's chorea (HC) is an autosomal dominant disorder so that at birth the risk that she had inherited the disease was 1 in 2. However, as she gets older, provided she remains unaffected, it becomes less and less likely that she is carrying the gene. By 53 years of age the risk has fallen to about 1 in 4 because only a third of individuals possessing the gene for HC have not developed the disorder by this age.*

b The risk is 1 in 8 for her son and 1 in 16 for each of her grandchildren.

c Huntington's chorea causes progressive chorea and dementia. No treatment halts the inexorable downhill course and death usually occurs about a decade after the onset of symptoms.

d A DNA marker which is closely linked to HC has recently been discovered and maps the locus to the short arm of chromosome 4. This marker and others under development offer the imminent prospect of presymptomatic and prenatal diagnosis in at least some HC families. (see questions 89 and 90).

---

*Consider six individuals at 1 in 2 risk at birth. On average, three will have inherited the HC gene and by 53 years of age two of them will have developed the disease. This leaves four asymptomatic individuals, one of whom will be carrying the disease gene.

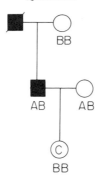

89 This is the pedigree of a family with Huntington's chorea showing
    the results of testing with a DNA marker (a restriction fragment
    length polymorphism with fragment patterns denoted by A and B
    detected by the DNA probe G8). This marker is closely linked to
    the HC locus on the short arm of chromosome 4 with a
    recombination fraction of about 5%. The consultand (C) is 20
    years of age and wishes to know the risk that she has inherited the
    gene for HC from her father.
    a What was the risk to the consultand before the DNA marker
       was studied?
    b What is the phase of disease and marker in the consultand's
       father?
    c What is the risk to the consultand given the results of the DNA
       marker?

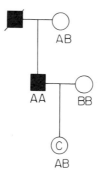

90 This is the pedigree of another family with Huntington's chorea
    studied with the same DNA marker as in the previous questions.
    a What is the risk to the consultand?

89   Huntington's chorea

  a 1 in 2. The risk is not significantly modified by her age because she is only 20 years old.

  b The consultand's father is heterozygous for the marker with the fragment pattern AB. Since his mother is homozygous BB, he must have inherited A along with the disease from his father who is known to have died from the condition. Therefore he has the HC gene and fragment pattern A together on one chromosome 4 and the corresponding normal gene and pattern B on the other.

  c About 1 in 20. She has received fragment pattern B from her father and will not have received the gene for Huntington's chorea unless a crossover has occurred. The chance of this happening is equal to the recombination fraction which is about 5%. The risk to the consultand's offspring would be approximately 1 in 40.

90   Huntington's chorea

  a 1 in 2. Her pedigree risk is unaltered because in this case her father is AA with the same fragment pattern on both of his chromosomes. The DNA marker is uninformative and cannot provide any information about the transmission of the disease to his daughter. Other DNA markers linked to the HC locus would have to be studied.

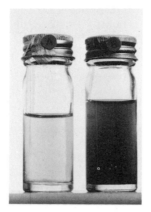

91 **A 40-year-old man is investigated for an arthropathy involving the spine, knees and hips. His urine turns brown on standing.**
   a What is the likely diagnosis?
   b How could this diagnosis be confirmed?
   c What is the prognosis?
   d What is the mode of inheritance?

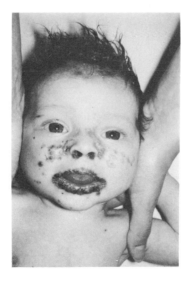

92 **This child was admitted for investigation of diarrhoea, failure to thrive and a skin eruption on the face, hands, feet and perineum.**
   a What is the likely diagnosis?
   b How may this diagnosis be confirmed?
   c What is the prognosis?
   d What is the recurrence risk?

91 a Alkaptonuria
   b The urine contains homogentisic acid.
   c Lifespan is normal.
   d Autosomal recessive trait due to deficiency of homogentisic acid oxidase.

92 Acrodermatitis enteropathica
   a This is the characteristic presentation and skin lesions of acrodermatitis enteropathica, a rare inherited disorder resulting in zinc deficiency. Some degree of alopecia is often present.
   b Plasma zinc is markedly reduced.
   c Untreated most children die before the age of 3 years. Treatment with oral zinc reverses all the clinical features.
   d This is an autosomal recessive trait with a 1 in 4 recurrence risk. Carrier detection is not possible. A phenocopy can be produced in the offspring of a mother with severe zinc deficiency.

93 **A woman develops rubella in the 12th week of pregnancy.**
   a What is the risk to her fetus?
   b What tests might be helpful?

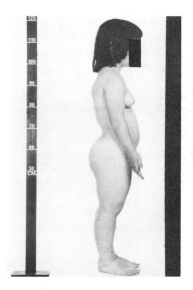

94 **This girl has disproportionate short stature with an upper to lower segment ratio of 1.3 (normal at her age 1.0). Her head circumference is normal.**
   a What is the likely diagnosis?
   b How may this diagnosis be confirmed?
   c What is the prognosis?
   d What is the mode of inheritance?

93   Congenital rubella
   a The frequency of fetal infection is 50% when a mother has
      rubella in the first trimester. Fetal infection may cause
      microcephaly, mental retardation, deafness, cataracts and
      congenital heart disease.
   b Fetal blood sampling is indicated at 18 weeks to test for fetal
      IgM specific for rubella. If present, termination of pregnancy
      should be considered.

94   Hypochondroplasia
   a Hypochondroplasia is the likeliest diagnosis with moderate
      short-limbed short stature and a normally shaped skull.
   b A skeletal survey will show characteristic but variable changes
      including: lack of caudal widening of the lumbar interpedicular
      distance; scalloping of the lumbar vertebrae on lateral view;
      distal prolongation of the fibula; prominence of muscle
      attachment sites.
   c Adult height within the range 48–60 inches (120–150 cm.).
      Intelligence and lifespan are usually normal.
   d Autosomal dominant.

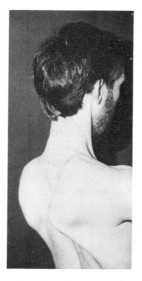

95 This 20-year-old man has facial weakness and foot drop. His father is asymptomatic but has mild facial weakness.
a What is the likely diagnosis?
b What are the clinical features of this disorder?
c How should the diagnosis be confirmed?
d What is the prognosis?
e Is prenatal diagnosis available?

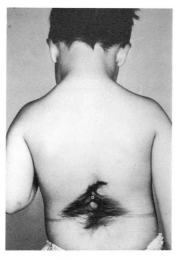

96 a What diagnosis should be considered?
b Is there an increased risk to subsequent offspring?

95 Facio-scapulo-humeral muscular dystrophy

a Facial weakness, wasting of the shoulder girdle muscles, winging of the scapulae and anterior tibial weakness is characteristic of facio-scapulo-humeral muscular dystrophy.

b Onset is usually in adolescence. Facial weakness results in expressionless facies with pouting lips. Wasting and weakness selectively involves the shoulder girdle and upper arm muscles. Anterior tibial weakness is often an early feature but involvement of proximal lower limb muscles occurs much later. Expression is very variable and the only manifestation may be facial weakness in individuals who are asymptomatic, as in the father in this example. Hence the importance of examining available relatives in apparently sporadic cases.

c EMG and muscle biopsy are indicated to confirm the diagnosis and exclude other myopathies and spinal muscular atrophy. Serum creatine kinase is normal or mildly elevated.

d Facio-scapulo-humeral muscular dystrophy usually follows a benign course with periods of apparent arrest and many patients experience little disability throughout a normal lifespan.

e Prenatal diagnosis is not available. Presymptomatic cases cannot be reliably identified either and do not have elevated levels of serum creatine kinase.

96 Spinal dysraphism

a A hairy patch of skin over the spine is often associated with spinal dysraphism. Neurological deficit may be present. X-ray would show widening of the vertebral canal and abnormalities of several vertebrae.

b Spinal dysraphism should be regarded as part of the spectrum of neural tube defects with a similar recurrence risk to anencephaly and spina bifida (see questions 58 and 68).

   The term spina bifida occulta is sometimes applied to this type of lesion. The same term is also used to describe the common incidental finding of a minor radiological defect in the neural arch of only one or two vertebrae which has no clinical significance.

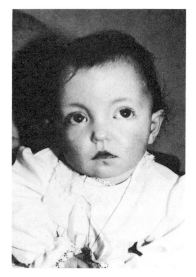

97 **This child is mentally retarded.**
   a What is the likely diagnosis?
   b How could this diagnosis be confirmed?
   c What is the prognosis?
   d What is the recurrence risk?

98 A couple attend for counselling with their first child who is
   congenitally deaf. The pregnancy was uneventful and screening
   for congenital infection is negative. The girl is otherwise normal
   and the parents are healthy and have normal hearing.
   a What is the incidence of congenital deafness?
   b What are the causes of congenital deafness?
   c What is the most likely cause of this child's deafness?
   d What is the recurrence risk?

97 Wolf syndrome

a Mental retardation with a Roman helmet appearance of the nasal bridge suggests the Wolf syndrome.

b Chromosome analysis will demonstrate partial deletion of the short arm of chromosome 4 (4p − syndrome).

c Mental retardation is profound and death usually occurs in early childhood.

d Parental chromosomes must be examined. If their chromosome are normal the recurrence risk is low. If one parent has a balanced translocation then the recurrence risk is about 20%.

98 Congenital deafness

a One in every 1000 children is congenitally deaf.

b Fifty per cent are due to a single gene disorder (87% autosomal recessive, 12% autosomal dominant, 1% X-linked recessive), 30% are environmental and 20% idiopathic.

c Probably genetic.

d The empiric recurrence risk for such couples is 1 in 6. This is the consequence of families with autosomal recessive deafness and a 1 in 4 risk being indistinguishable from those where the deafness is idiopathic or due to a new dominant mutation with a low recurrence risk. If this couple should have another deaf child the diagnosis is almost certainly autosomal recessive deafness and the recurrence risk would increase to 1 in 4 for subsequent offspring.

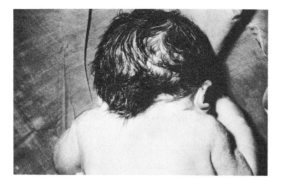

99 **a** What is the diagnosis?
     b What other features may be associated?
     c What is the mode of inheritance?

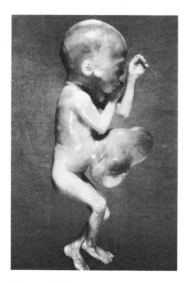

100 **a** What is the diagnosis?
      b Why is chromosome analysis indicated?
      c What is the prognosis?
      d What is the recurrence risk?
      e Is prenatal diagnosis available?

99 Klippel–Feil syndrome

a Klippel-Feil syndrome with short stiff neck due to fusion of the cervical vertebrae.

b Congenital heart disease (25%), renal malformations (30%) and Sprengel deformity (hypoplastic elevated scapula).

c This is a sporadic disorder with a low recurrence risk.

100 Exomphalos

a Exomphalos: an anterior abdominal wall defect involving the umbilical cord and enclosed in a sac (syn. omphalocele).

b Thirty per cent of cases are associated with chromosome abnormalities, especially trisomy 13 or 18.

c Surgical correction is possible.

d Isolated exomphalos has a low recurrence risk.

e Prenatal diagnosis is possible by ultrasound. These lesions cause elevated maternal serum alphafetoprotein and will usually be detected in screening programmes for neural tube defects. Amniocentesis is indicated to exclude an associated chromosome abnormality.

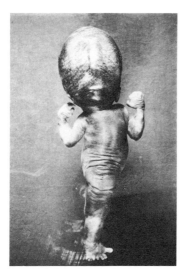

101 **a** What is the diagnosis?
          b What other features may occur?
          c What is the prognosis?
          d What is the recurrence risk?

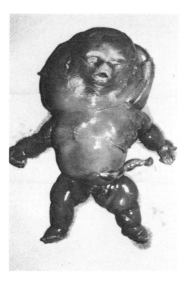

102 **This fetus was spontaneously miscarried at 23 weeks gestation.**
          a What diagnosis should be suspected?
          b How could this diagnosis be confirmed?

101 a Sirenomelia.
   b Associated features include lower vertebral defects, single
      umbilical artery, urogenital anomalies and variable leg
      malformations.
   c The prognosis is generally poor because of the associated renal
      problems.
   d This is a sporadic malformation with a low recurrence risk.

102 Turner's syndrome
   a This female fetus has marked nuchal swellings (cystic hygroma)
      suggesting Turner's syndrome. Ninety nine per cent of all
      conceptions with 45,X miscarry spontaneously.
   b Fibroblasts can be cultured from skin or fascia lata (even 1−3
      days after death) and karyotyped to confirm 45, X.

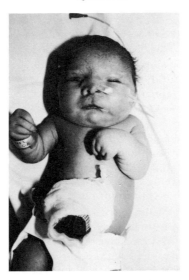

103 **This infant was small for gestational age. A routine chromosome analysis on a peripheral blood sample was normal.**
   a What diagnosis should be considered?
   b How may this be confirmed?
   c What is the prognosis?
   d What is the recurrence risk?

104 **A male Chinese infant has prologed jaundice and his mother comments that her brother had the same problem.**
   a What is the likely diagnosis?
   b How may this diagnosis be confirmed?
   c What is the mode of inheritance?
   d What is the prognosis?

103   Trisomy 18 mosaic
   a The combination of exomphalos, flexed overlapping digits and
      facial dysmorphology suggests trisomy 18.
   b A normal blood chromosome analysis does not exclude
      mosaicism and if the clinical findings are strongly suggestive of
      a chromosome abnormality the chromosomes should be
      examined in a second blood sample and also skin fibroblasts. In
      this child mosaicism for trisomy 18 was demonstrated.
   c The prognosis depends on which tissues are involved and the
      proportion of cells which are abnormal.
   d The recurrence risk for chromosomal mosaicism in sibs is very
      low.

104   a Glucose-6-phosphate dehydrogenase (G6PD) deficiency.
   b Quantitative and qualitative assay of G6PD in red blood cells.
   c This is an X-linked recessive disorder with the locus at the tip
      of the long arm of the X-chromosome. More than 150 molecular
      variants of this enzyme are known (multiple allelism). Glucose-
      6-phosphate dehydrogenase deficiency is common in
      Mediterranean, Middle Eastern, African and Oriental ethnic
      groups. If the gene frequency is sufficiently high homozygous
      females with G6PD will be encountered (for example, in
      American blacks 13% of males and 2% of females are affected).
   d Deficiency of G6PD impairs the ability of the red cell to
      maintain haemoglobin in the reduced state. Most affected
      individuals are asymptomatic until exposed to oxidant drugs
      (sulphonamides and antimalarials), broad beans (favism) or
      infection, all of which can precipitate an acute haemolytic crisis.
      This is usually self-limiting and followed by recovery even if
      exposure continues. The deficiency is predominantly in older
      red cells (it is the stability of the enzyme which appears to be
      defective) and as the marrow responds these are replaced by
      young red cells with higher enzyme levels which resist
      oxidation. Sometimes G6PD deficiency is associated with a
      chronic haemolytic anaemia. Family members at risk should be
      screened and counselled.

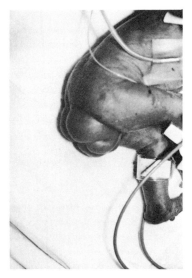

105 **This child has several fingers missing from one hand.**
    a What is the abnormality shown and what is the diagnosis?
    b What other features may be present?
    c What is the recurrence risk?

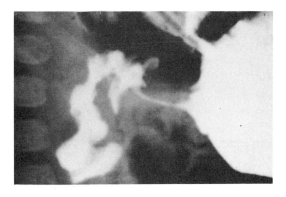

106 **This is the X-ray of a 4-week-old infant.**
    a What is the diagnosis?
    b What is the mode of inheritance?
    c What is the recurrence risk?

105   Amniotic bands
   a   Constriction and distal oedema of the buttocks due to amniotic
       bands which would also be responsible for amputation of the
       fingers.
   b   Premature rupture of the amnion is believed to result in bands
       which may encircle and disrupt portions of the fetus. Features
       tend to be asymmetric and vary from case to case but include
       transverse limb defects, distal pseudosyndactyly,
       craniostenosis, unusual facial clefts and thoracic or abdominal
       wall defects.
   c   This is usually a sporadic disorder with a low recurrence risk.

106   a   Hypertrophic pyloric stenosis.
   b   Pyloric stenosis is inherited as a multifactoral trait. It is much
       commoner in males than females (5:1) and so the recurrence risk
       depends on the sex of the index case.
   c   If a male child is affected the recurrence risk is 1 in 30 whereas
       for a female index case the recurrence risk is 1 in 15.

107 **A 38-year-old woman requests counselling before undertaking her
first pregnancy.**
   a What are the genetic risks to be considered?
   b What investigation may be indicated?
   c What are the risks of the test itself?

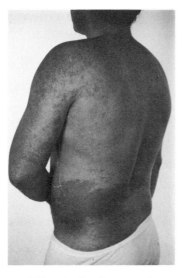 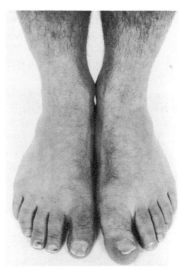

108 **a** What is the diagnosis?
   b What other features may be present?
   c What is the prognosis?
   d What is the recurrence risk?

109 **A woman with multiple sclerosis requests genetic counselling.**
   a What is the risk of multiple sclerosis in her offspring?
   b Is prenatal diagnosis available?
   c What else should be mentioned?

107 Maternal age
  a The risk of chromosome abnormalities, especially trisomy 21
     (Down syndrome) increases with advancing maternal age. At 38
     years of age the birth incidence is 1 in 100 (1 in 200 for trisomy
     21 alone).
  b Amniocentesis at 16–17 weeks gestation and fetal chromosome
     analysis should be offered. The chance of finding a chromosome
     abnormality in this woman would be 1 in 60, higher than at
     birth because of the substantial fetal loss rate for such
     pregnancies between 16 weeks and term.
  c The risk of miscarriage following amniocentesis is 1 in 300 in
     major obstetric units.

108 Klippel–Trenaunay–Weber syndrome
  a The combination of limb overgrowth and vascular naevi is
     typical of the Klippel–Trenaunay–Weber syndrome.
  b Venous varicosities, pigmented naevi, arteriovenous fistulas,
     macrocephaly, visceromegaly and asymmetric facial
     hypertrophy.
  c Disproportionate growth of a limb may rarely require
     amputation. Mental retardation can occur. Malignant change is
     not a feature.
  d This is a sporadic disorder with a low recurrence risk.

109 Multiple sclerosis
  a In the United Kingdom the frequency of multiple sclerosis is
     1 in 2000 and the risk to sibs and offspring is 1 in 100.
  b Prenatal diagnosis is not possible.
  c On average 1 in 5 women will relapse during or soon after
     pregnancy which is double the rate in non-pregnant women.

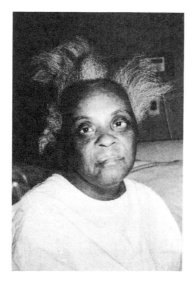

110   This 60-year-old woman is mentally retarded.
   a   What is the diagnosis?
   b   How may this diagnosis be confirmed?
   c   What complication may occur at this age?

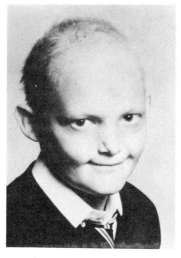

111   This boy has no teeth.
   a   What is the diagnosis?
   b   What is the prognosis?
   c   What is the mode of inheritance?

110   Down's syndrome

   a Down's syndrome. The facial features in adults are less marked than in childhood.

   b Chromosome analysis to confirm the presence of an additional chromosome 21.

   c Presenile dementia is very common in older patients with Down's syndrome.

111   Hypohidrotic ectodermal dysplasia

   a The sparse hair and depressed nasal bridge are characteristic of hypohidrotic ectodermal dysplasia. Reduced or absent sweat glands and partial or complete anodontia are consistent features.

   b Hyperthermia due to inadequate sweating can be a threat to life, especially in early childhood. Respiratory tract infections are common.

   c This is inherited as an X-linked recessive trait. The female carriers may show hypodontia, sparse hair and a reduced dermal ridge pore count or a patchy pattern of sweating.

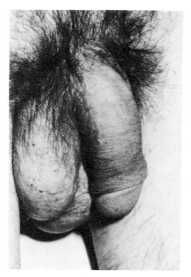

112 This man has suffered repeated episodes of fever and excruciating
pain in the extremities since childhood. His mother died of renal
failure at 50 years of age. The tiny lesions on his scrotum are
purple in colour.

   a What is the likely diagnosis?

   b How may this diagnosis be confirmed?

   c What is the mode of inheritance?

   d Is family screening indicated?

113 A woman with achondroplasia presents in the 16th week of her
first pregnancy. Her husband also has achondroplasia.

   a What are the risks to the pregnancy?

   b Is prenatal diagnosis possible?

114 A woman develops chickenpox in the 14th week of pregnancy.

   a What is the risk for her fetus?

   b Will any tests be helpful?

112 **Fabry disease**

   a This is the typical history of Fabry disease and the picture shows the characteristic angiokeratomas over the scrotum. Other common sites are the buttocks, inguinal and umbilical areas. The lesions are 1−3 mm diameter purple to blue-black papules which may have a hyperkeratotic surface.

   b Proteinuria and other evidence of renal impairment may be present and slit-lamp examination will show corneal opacities. Absence of leucocyte alpha-galactosidase activity confirms the diagnosis.

   c X-linked recessive.

   d Family screening is indicated because this is a serious disorder causing renal or cardiac failure in males in middle adult life. Female carriers manifest the condition to a variable extent but can sometimes be severely affected as in this example. Carrier detection depends on the demonstration of two populations of hair root bulbs, one with deficient alpha-galactosidase and the other with normal enzyme levels, corresponding to inactivation of the normal and carrier X chromosomes respectively.

113 **Achondroplasia**

   a It is important to confirm the diagnosis. If both have achondroplasia then on average a quarter of their children will be unaffected, half will have achondroplasia and a quarter will have homozygous achondroplasia. The latter results in extreme bony shortening and death in the neonatal period. Apart from these genetic risks a Caesarian section will be required in view of the small maternal pelvis.

   b Prenatal diagnosis is possible with serial measurements of fetal long bone lengths using ultrasound. Heterozygous achondroplasia is apparent by the end of the second trimester; homozygous achondroplasia is apparent earlier.

114 **Fetal varicella**

   a There is a risk of fetal varicella with chorioretinitis, mental retardation, seizures and cutaneous scars. The frequency of fetal infection and the most critical period are unknown.

   b Fetal blood sampling to demonstrate IgM specific for varicella is indicated.

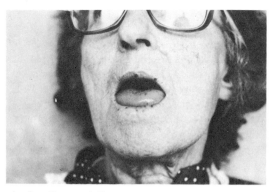

115 a What is the diagnosis?
     b What is the prognosis?
     c What is the mode of inheritance?

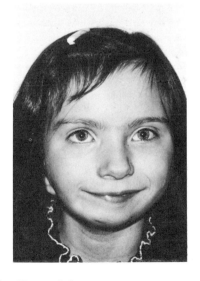

116 a What is the diagnosis?
     b What other features may be found?
     c What is the prognosis?
     d What is the recurrence risk?

115 Hereditary haemorrhagic telangiectasia

a The lesions on the lips are characteristic of hereditary haemorrhagic telangiectasia (Osler–Weber–Rendu disease). These clusters of telangiectatic blood vessels appear at puberty as red/purple macules or papules, most commonly on the lips, tongue and nasal mucosa.

b Bleeding may occur from the nose, mouth, lungs, gastrointestinal and urinary tracts and can be severe. Recurrent epistaxis may be improved by oestrogen therapy to induce squamous metaplasia of nasal mucous membranes. Pulmonary arteriovenous fistulae and hepatic cirrhosis may occur.

c Autosomal dominant.

116 Hemifacial microsomia

a This girl has hemifacial microsomia (note the position of the right ear).

b Asymmetric maldevelopment of structures from the first and second branchial arches including microtia, preauricular tags, conductive deafness and diminished parotid secretion. If ocular and vertebral anomalies are present then the term Goldenhar syndrome may be applied.

c Occasionally mental retardation is present. Otherwise the prognosis is good.

d Usually sporadic with a low recurrence risk.

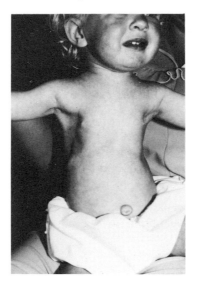

117 **This 2-year-old girl had severe respiratory difficulties in infancy.**
   a What is the likely diagnosis?
   b How may this diagnosis be confirmed?
   c What is the prognosis?
   d What is the mode of inheritance?

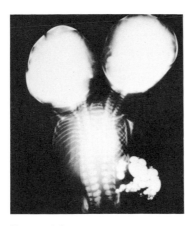

118 **a** What is the diagnosis?
   b What is the aetiology?
   c What is the prognosis?
   d What is the recurrence risk?

117 a **Jeunes asphyxiating thoracic dysplasia.**

  b Radiological features include a narrow bell-shaped thorax and abnormal pelvis with a spiky acetabular roof. Limb shortening is variable. Similar radiographic features occur in chondroectodermal dysplasia (Ellis–van Creveld syndrome) but these children have characteristic gingival abnormalities (see question 84).

  c Death in the newborn period due to respiratory insufficiency is common. In surviving children the respiratory problems diminish with age, but renal failure often develops in adolescence or early adult life.

  d Autosomal recessive.

118 a **Conjoined twins.**

  b Incomplete separation occurs in about 1% of monozygotic twins.

  c The commonest type is thoracopagus (joined at the thorax) but juncture at the head, buttocks or elsewhere may be seen. Ten to twenty per cent have other malformations and the prognosis depends upon these and the extent of shared organs.

  d Negligible.

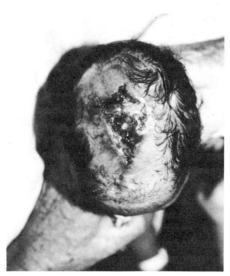

119 **This is the scalp of a neonate who had an uneventful gestation and delivery.**
  a What is the diagnosis?
  b What is the aetiology?
  c What is the prognosis?
  d What is the recurrence risk?

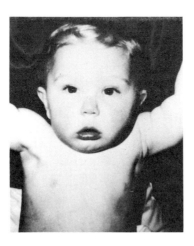

120 **a** What is the diagnosis?
  b What other features may be associated?
  c What is the prognosis?
  d What is the recurrence risk?

119 **a** **Aplasia cutis congenita.**
    b This may be primary (sporadic or familial) but is also a characteristic feature of trisomy 13.
    c The skin defect heals with scarring and alopecia.
    d Familial cases show autosomal dominant inheritance.

120 **Poland syndrome**
    a Unilateral absence of the pectoralis muscle is a cardinal feature of the Poland syndrome.
    b Ipsilateral hand syndactyly.
    c Normal intelligence and lifespan.
    d This is a sporadic defect with a low recurrence risk.

121   A neonate has dysphagia and bilateral palsies of the sixth and
      seventh cranial nerves.
      a   What is the likely diagnosis?
      b   What other features may be present?
      c   What is the prognosis?
      d   What is the recurrence risk?

122   A woman presents at 13 weeks gestation in her first pregnancy
      concerned about the risk to the baby in view of a family history of
      Hurler syndrome. This diagnosis was made in her brother who
      died at the age of 18 years. Scrutiny of the hospital records shows
      that he had progressive intellectual deterioration, short stature,
      coarse facial features, clear corneas, hepatosplenomegaly and
      excess dermatan and heparan sulphate in the urine.
      a   What is the risk to her pregnancy?
      b   Are any investigations indicated?

123   A 3-year-old boy is investigated for progessive ataxia. His serum
      alphafetoprotein is grossly elevated.
      a   What is the likely diagnosis?
      b   What other features may be present?
      c   What is the prognosis?
      d   What is the mode of inheritance?

121 Moebius syndome.

   a Moebius syndrome is the most likely diagnosis. The usual pathological finding is aplasia of the sixth and seventh cranial nerve nuclei. Congenital myotonic dystrophy should be considered in the differential diagnosis.

   b Micrognathia and talipes are common. Other cranial nerves may be involved including the hypoglossal causing fasciculation of the tongue.

   c About 15% are mentally retarded and death in infancy is usual in the severely affected individuals.

   d Usually sporadic with a low recurrence risk.

122 Hunter syndrome

   a Hurler syndrome is autosomal recessive and the risk to the pregnancy would be very small if this was the diagnosis. However, absence of corneal clouding and survival to 18 years of age makes Hunter syndrome the likely diagnosis. This is an X-linked recessive disorder and poses a significant risk to the pregnancy.

   b Carriers for Hunter syndrome can be identified by assay of iduronate sulphate sulphatase in serum and hair roots. In this case both the consultand and her mother were shown to be carriers. Following amniocentesis at 16 weeks gestation the fetus was found to be male and prenatal diagnosis by two-dimensional electrophoresis of glycosaminoglycans (GAGS) in amniotic fluid and by specific enzyme assay in cultured amniotic fluid cells showed the presence of Hunter syndrome.

123 Ataxia telangiectasia

   a The combination of progressive ataxia with elevated AFP is characteristic of ataxia telangiectasia.

   b Telangiectasia of bulbar conjunctiva, nasal bridge and pinnae are typical in later childhood. IgA may be reduced. Spontaneous chromosome breakage is increased but the diagnostic cytogenetic finding is the profound sensitivity of cultured skin fibroblasts to X-irradiation.

   c Immune deficiency results in recurrent infection and 10% develop malignancy. The neurological defects are progressive and death usually occurs in late childhood.

   d This is inherited as an autosomal recessive trait. Carrier detection is not possible but prenatal diagnosis has been achieved by demonstrating excessive radiosensitivity of cultured amniotic fluid cells.

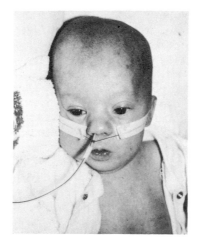

124 This infant has wide cranial sutures with a large anterior fontanelle, hypotonia and hepatomegaly.
  a What is the likely diagnosis?
  b How may this diagnosis be confirmed?
  c What is the prognosis?
  d What is the recurrence risk?

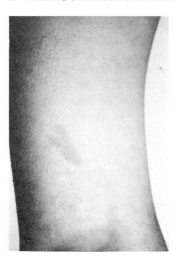 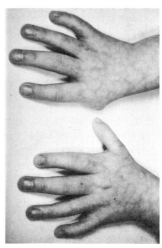

125 This 8-year-old girl has normocytic anaemia, leucopenia and thrombocytopenia.
  a What is the likely diagnosis?
  b How would this diagnosis be confirmed?
  c What is the mode of inheritance?
  d What is the prognosis?

124   Zellweger syndrome
  a   The high forehead, wide sutures and large fontanelle, hypotonia
      and hepatomegaly suggest Zellweger syndrome (cerebro-hepato-
      renal syndrome). Other features which may be present
      include redundant skin over the nape of the neck and
      contractures. This clinical appearance can be confused with
      trisomy 21.
  b   Serum iron is increased, liver function tests are abnormal and
      the urine contains pipecolic acid. Plasma long chain fatty acids
      are increased and current evidence indicates a primary defect in
      peroxisomes.
  c   Most affected children die in infancy. Autopsy shows renal
      cysts and excessive iron in the liver with portal fibrosis.
  d   This is an autosomal recessive disorder with a 1 in 4 recurrence
      risk. Carrier detection is not possible. Prenatal diagnosis has
      been achieved by assay of long chain fatty acids in cultured
      amniotic fluid cells.

125   Fanconi anaemia
  a   *Cafe au lait* spots and hyperpigmentation, radial defects (in this
      case hypoplasia of the left thumb and aplasia of the right) and
      pancytopenia are characteristic of Fanconi anaemia. Short
      stature is common. The limb defect can be more extensive with
      hypoplasia or absence of the radius. Other congenital
      abnormalities are often present, particularly renal anomalies.
  b   Chromosome analysis shows an increased frequency of
      spontaneous chromosome breakage. The bone marrow is
      hypoplastic. Fetal haemoglobin may be elevated.
  c   This is an autosomal recessive disorder and is often associated
      with parental consanguinity.
  d   Life expectancy is reduced. The commonest complications result
      from pancytopenia but these patients also have an increased
      susceptibility to malignancy, especially leukaemias and
      lymphomas.

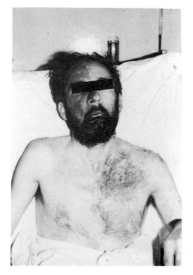

126 **This man has epilepsy.**
    a What is the likely diagnosis?
    b What tests would confirm the diagnosis?
    c What are the complications?
    d What is the mode of inheritance?

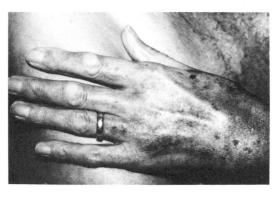

127 **This middle-aged lady complains of hirsutism.**
    a What is the likely diagnosis?
    b How could this diagnosis be confirmed?
    c What is the mode of inheritance?

126   Sturge—Weber syndrome
   a The capillary haemangioma (port wine stain) in the distribution
      of the right trigeminal nerve is typical of the Sturge—Weber
      syndrome.
   b Skull X-ray would demonstrate calcification around an
      ipsilateral pia-arachnoid vascular malformation. This develops
      during childhood and is present in the majority of adults.
   c Cortical damage secondary to the vascular malformation can
      result in seizures, mental retardation and hemiparesis on the
      contralateral side. Haemangioma of the choriod can cause
      buphthalmos or glaucoma.
   d This is a sporadic disorder and there is no increased risk to his
      offspring.

127   Porphyria cutanea tarda
   a The combination of hirsutism, pigmentation of exposed areas
      and white blisters over the knuckles suggests porphyria cutanea
      tarda.
   b The urine contains increased uroporphyrinogen III and there
      are increased fecal porphyrins. Red cell uroporphyrinogen
      decarboxylase is reduced in the familial form.
   c Most cases are sporadic and associated with liver disease or
      exposure to drugs or alcohol. The familial form is autosomal
      dominant.

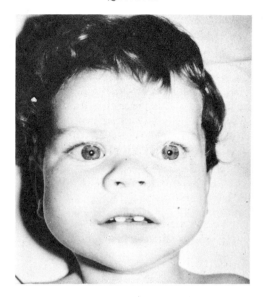

128 **This boy has supravalvular aortic stenosis.**
  a What is the diagnosis?
  b What other features may be found?
  c What is the recurrence risk?

129 **A young man is admitted for repair of an inguinal hernia. As a child he had a general anaesthetic for an appendicectomy, but nevertheless is worried because his father died under general anaesthesia.**
  a What diagnosis should be considered?
  b How can this diagnosis be confirmed?
  c What is the prognosis?
  d What is the mode of inheritance?

128 Williams syndrome
  a This is the characteristic facies of the Williams syndrome with prominent upper lips and a small anteverted nose. Supravalvular aortic stenosis is a common feature of this condition.
  b Short stature, mental retardation (usually mild) and transient hypercalcaemia.
  c This is a sporadic disorder with a low recurrence risk.

129 Hyperthermia of anaesthesia
  a The family history raises the possibility of hyperthermia of anaesthesia (malignant hyperpyrexia) and more information about the circumstances of his father's death should be sought. Previous uneventful general anaesthesia does not exclude the diagnosis.
  b The creatine phosphokinase may be elevated but definitive diagnosis requires muscle biopsy and *in vitro* exposure of muscle tissue to trigger agents.
  c Suxamethonium or halothane trigger explosive hyperpyrexia and hypertonia with a 60% mortality.
  d Autosomal dominant. Family members at risk should be screened and those found to have the disorder should carry a warning card.

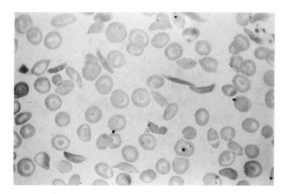

130 Blood film from an African child.
  a What is the likely diagnosis and how is this confirmed?
  b What is the basic genetic defect?
  c Is carrier detection possible?
  d What is the recurrence risk?
  e Is prenatal diagnosis possible?

131 A newborn male with seizures has the following biochemical profile: plasma glucose 2.5 mmol/l (45 gm/dl), plasma calcium 1.0 mmol/l (4 mg/dl) and plasma magnesium 0.8 mmol/l (2 mg/dl). A chest X-ray shows absence of the thymic shadow.
  a What diagnosis should be considered?
  b What is the pathophysiology?
  c What is the prognosis?
  d What is the recurrence risk?

130 Sickle cell disease

a The red cells have the characteristic sickled shape seen in sickle cell disease. Haemoglobin electrophoresis shows 85−95% haemoglobin S with haemoglobin F making up the total.

b A point mutation in the sixth codon of the beta globin gene on chromosome 11 substitutes valine for glutamic acid at this position. The resulting HbS has a different electrophoretic mobility from HbA. At reduced oxygen tension HbS molecules form rod-like aggregates which distort the red cell.

c Carriers (heterozygotes) have one sickle gene and one normal beta globin gene. This can be demonstrated by haemoglobin electrophoresis which will show 30−45% HbS with HbA making up the total. At these concentrations of HbS sickling only occurs with severe hypoxia such as might result from shock or high altitude.

d Both parents must be carriers. The risk of another affected child homozygous for the sickle gene is 1 in 4.

e Prenatal diagnosis is possible by analysis of fetal DNA obtained by chorionic villus sampling or amniocentesis. The point mutation causing the disease abolishes a restriction enzyme recognition site and results in an altered pattern of fragments after DNA digestion.

131 DiGeorge syndrome

a The seizures are due to hypocalcaemia and absence of the thymic shadow suggests DiGeorge syndrome.

b Abnormal development of the third and fourth pharyngeal pouches results in deficiency of the thymus and parathyroid glands. Lack of parathyroid hormone is responsible for hypocalcaemia. Cell-mediated immunity is impaired resulting in recurrent viral and fungal infections and failure to thrive. Immunoglobulins are usually normal. There may be associated cardiac and aortic arch anomalies.

c Many affected infants die from immunodeficiency or from aortic arch abnormalities. Thymic transplantation is sometimes successful.

d Usually sporadic with a low recurrence risk. Some patients have shown an interstitial microdeletion of chromosome 22 and one family has been described where recurrence occurred and a parent had a balanced structural rearrangement of chromosome 22. Detailed prometaphase chromosome studies of infants with DiGeorge syndrome are therefore indicated.

132 A male neonate is transferred to the intensive care unit at 36 hours
of age with a 24 hour history of increasing lethargy and
hypotonia. Pregnancy and delivery had been uneventful. A
brother died at one week of age with similar symptoms.
   a What is the differential diagnosis?
   b What investigations are required?

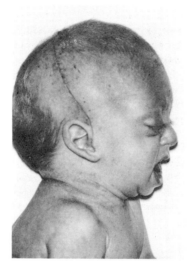

133 a What is the likely diagnosis?
   b What is the prognosis?
   c What is the mode of inheritance?

132   Ornithine transcarbamylase deficiency

a The major differential diagnoses are sepsis and an inborn error of metabolism.

b The baby should be screened for infection. Biochemical investigation on the blood should include urea and electrolytes, acid-base status, ammonia, glucose and amino acid profile. Urine should be obtained for amino acid and organic acid profiles.

In this case pronounced hyperammonaemia was present but no specific abnormality of the plasma amino acid pattern. This suggested a urea cycle enzyme defect, of which ornithine transcarbamylase (OTC) deficiency is the most common, and strong supporting evidence for this came from the finding of gross orotic aciduria. The definitive diagnosis was made by demonstrating deficiency of hepatic ornithine transcarbamylase.

133   Crouzon syndrome

a The combination of acrocephaly due to craniosynostosis, proptosis due to shallow orbits and a parrot-like nose is typical of Crouzon syndrome (craniofacial dysostosis). The hands are normal in this syndrome. Compare with Apert syndrome (question 38).

b The degree of craniostenosis is variable and surgical decompression is necessary in the more severe cases to permit normal brain development.

c Autosomal dominant, but with variable expression so that it is important to examine the parents carefully before concluding that an affected child represents a fresh mutation.

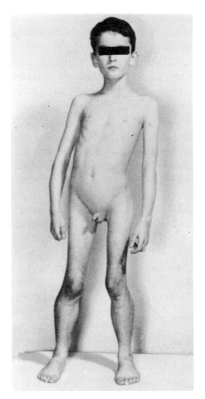

134 This boy presented with a waddling gait at 3 years of age and is unable to climb stairs or get up from the floor unaided at the age of 8 years. He has a serum creatine kinase of 4300 IU/l. He is an only child and there is no family history of this condition. His mother's creatine kinase on three separate estimations was 80, 76 and 84 IU/l. (Upper limit of normal in females: 91 IU/l).

a What is the likely diagnosis?
b What is the prognosis?
c What would be the risk of another affected child?
d What tests (if any) should be offered in a future pregnancy?

134   Duchenne muscular dystrophy

a   The combination of proximal muscle wasting in the lower
limbs, lumbar lordosis and calf pseudohypertrophy in a boy
with massively elevated serum creatine kinase (CK) is typical of
Duchenne muscular dystrophy. EMG and muscle biopsy would
confirm the diagnosis. The age at onset and rapid progression
excludes Becker muscular dystrophy.

b   Muscular weakness is progressive. Most boys are chair-bound
by 10–12 years and die of pneumonia or heart failure at around
20 years of age.

c   Duchenne muscular dystrophy is an X-linked recessive
disorder, but a third of isolated cases are thought to represent
new mutations, so that in the absence of other information the
recurrence risk is not 1 in 4 but 1 in 6 ($\frac{2}{3} \times \frac{1}{4}$). About two
thirds of carrier women have CK levels within the normal
range. If the level is low normal, the chance that a woman is a
carrier may be substantially reduced. If the CK is in the upper
part of the normal range, as in this case, the risk is unchanged
or may actually be increased.

d   In view of this high risk the mother might seek prenatal
diagnosis by fetal sexing after chorionic villus sampling or
amniocentesis with termination of a male pregnancy. Recent
developments in molecular genetics have localized the gene for
Duchenne muscular dystrophy to the short arm of the X
chromosome and in certain families this technology can be used
for both carrier detection and prenatal diagnosis (see question
11).

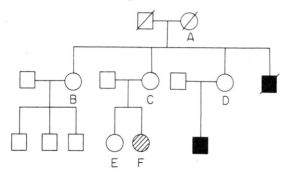

135 This is a family in which two boys have been affected by Duchenne muscular dystrophy. Female F has proximal muscle weakness, short stature and a serum creatine kinase of 3670 IU/l at 7 years of age.
a Which females are obligate carriers?
b Why might female F be affected with Duchenne muscular dystrophy?

136 A couple request counselling in view of the wife's grand mal epilepsy which is well controlled on sodium valproate.
a What is the risk of epilepsy in their offspring?
b What risks does her medication pose for her offspring?
c What tests (if any) are indicated during pregnancy?

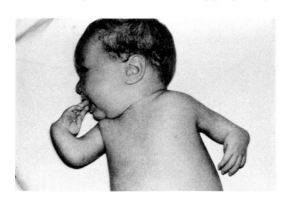

137 This neonate has bruising due to thrombocytopaenia.
a What is the likely diagnosis?
b How could this diagnosis be confirmed?
c What is the prognosis?
d What is the mode of inheritance?

135 Duchenne muscular dystrophy

a A and D are obligate carriers. C is also an obligate carrier if the EMG and muscle biopsy confirm that F has Duchenne muscular dystrophy. In this event E has a 1 in 2 chance of being a carrier. For B the chance of being a carrier is less than 1 in 2 because she has had three normal sons. When this is taken into account her chance of being a carrier works out to be 1 in 9. For both B and E creatine kinase levels should also be taken into account in calculating their final carrier risks.

b Duchenne muscular dystrophy is an X-linked recessive trait but carrier females may be mildly affected if by chance it is predominantly the normal X chromosomes which are inactivated in their muscle cells (manifesting heterozygote due to atypical lyonization). Theoretically a carrier female could have a new mutation at the same locus on her other X chromosome but this is extemely unlikely. Alternatively a woman with 45, X or monosomy for the short arm of the X chromosome would not inactivate the X chromosome carrying the mutant allele and would be as severely affected as a male.

In this family F had a high risk of inheriting the DMD allele and is as severely affected as a male. She is also short and chromosome analysis revealed 45, X.

136 Grand mal epilepsy

a The frequency of grand mal epilepsy in the general population is 1 in 200. The frequency in the offspring of this couple will be 1 in 25.

b Epileptic mothers on anticonvulsant therapy have an increased risk of congenital malformations in their offspring. Sodium valproate is not safer than other anticonvulsants in this respect and the risk of a major malformation is probably doubled to 6% with cleft lip and palate and neural tube defects amongst the specifically associated lesions.

c Screening for neural tube defects by serial ultrasound scanning and amniocentesis for alphafetoprotein assay should be considered.

137 TAR syndrome

a The combination of thrombocytopaenia with bilateral radial aplasia and preservation of the thumbs is typical of the TAR syndrome (Thrombocytopaenia–Absent Radius syndrome). In radial aplasia associated with other syndromes such as Holt-Oram syndrome the thumb is usually hypoplastic or absent.

b Radiographs confirm the hypoplasia or absence of the radii and bone marrow shows absent or reduced megakaryocytes.

138 **A couple request counselling because the man had a bilateral cleft lip and palate.**
   a How is cleft lip and palate inherited?
   b What is the risk of recurrence in their offspring?

139 **A woman has an intravenous pyelogram before it is realized that she is six weeks pregnant.**
   a What risks does irradiation pose for the fetus?
   b At what level of irradiation do these risks become apparent?
   c What tests are indicated during the pregnancy?

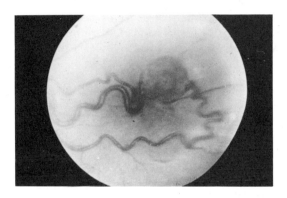

140 **This patient has a renal tumour and polycythaemia.**
   a What is the diagnosis?
   b What is the prognosis?
   c What is the mode of inheritance?

---

continued from p. 146.

   c About 40% die in infancy from haemorrhagic complications. Later the bleeding tendency usually improves. About 7% are mentally retarded.
   d Autosomal recessive. Carrier detection is not possible but prenatal diagnosis is possible by ultrasonic demonstration of the radial defects.

138 **Cleft lip and palate**

a Cleft lip and palate is inherited as a multifactorial trait. This infers that multiple genes at different loci must summate with environmental factors to produce the malformation. Thus within affected families the frequency is higher than the general population frequency. The pedigree pattern alone is not diagnostic of multifactorial inheritance and this conclusion is reached from combined family and twin studies. Cleft lip and palate may also be a feature of at least 100 syndromes and it is important to exclude these before counselling.

b For this couple with non-syndromic isolated cleft lip and palate the recurrence risk in their offspring is 1 in 20. If the lesion had been a unilateral cleft lip and palate in the husband the recurrence risk would have been lower (1 in 50).

139 **Irradiation**

a Fetal irradiation can cause congenital malformations, particularly microcephaly with mental retardation and an increased risk of childhood malignancy, especially leukaemia.

b An accidental diagnostic X-ray of one rad or less during early pregnancy results in an additional risk of fetal abnormality of 0.1%. With increasing doses the risk goes up proportionately and termination is usually advised if a fetus less than 8 weeks is exposed to more than 25 rads.

c An intravenous pyelogram results in a fetal dose of irradiation of less than one rad. The added risk to the pregnancy is extremely low and no special prenatal tests are indicated.

140 **von Hippel–Lindau disease**

a The combination of renal tumour and retinal haemangioma is characteristic of von Hippel–Lindau disease. Polycythaemia may be secondary to the renal tumour or to a coexistent cerebellar haemangioblastoma. Renal, pancreatic, hepatic and epididymal cysts may also occur.

b The cerebellar tumours are amenable to surgery. Renal carcinoma occurs in 20% and regular follow-up with abdominal CT scans is indicated in these patients.

c Autosomal dominant with variable expression. Prenatal diagnosis is not available.

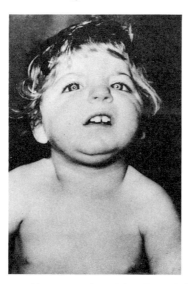

141 This child is mentally retarded and has broad thumbs and great toes.
   a What is the diagnosis?
   b What is the prognosis?
   c What is the recurrence risk?
   d Is prenatal diagnosis available?

142 A 12-year-old boy presents with renal colic. He is otherwise healthy. His urine gives a positive cyanide-nitroprusside test.
   a What is the likely diagnosis?
   b How may this diagnosis be confirmed?
   c What is the management?
   d What is the mode of inheritance?

143 A 25-year-old woman seeks genetic advice because her brother has motor neurone disease and this disorder also affected her mother and maternal grandfather.
   a What is the usual mode of inheritance of motor neurone disease?
   b What is the consultand's risk of developing this condition?

141   Rubinstein–Taybi syndrome
a Downslanting palpebral fissures with maxillary hypoplasia, broad thumbs and great toes are typical of the Rubinstein-Taybi syndrome.
b The degree of mental retardation is variable but most are moderately retarded.
c The recurrence risk appears to be low.
d Prenatal diagnosis is not possible.

142   Cystinuria
a A positive nitroprusside test occurs in homocystinuria, acetonuria and cystinuria. Only the last of these is associated with renal colic.
b Urinary amino acid chromatography confirms excessive excretion of cystine, arginine, ornithine and lysine. Cystine is relatively insoluble and produces radio-opaque calculi. Flat hexagonal shaped crystals of cystine are usually visible on urine microscopy.
c Untreated recurrent urolithiasis can result in renal failure. The objective of treatment is to keep the urine dilute and alkaline by maintaining a high fluid intake by day *and* by night and taking sodium citrate or bicarbonate. If these measures are not sufficient to prevent stone formation, D-penicillamine may be considered.
d Autosomal recessive.

143   Motor neurone disease
a Motor neurone disease (MND) is usually a sporadic disorder with a risk to first degree relatives of less than 1%.
b Hereditary motor neurone disease is a well documented entity with most families showing autosomal dominant inheritance as here. The clinical features are indistinguishable from the more common sporadic type. The risk that this young woman has inherited the disease gene is 1 in 2 but her risk of developing MND may well be lower than this because non-penetrance has been observed in some families giving rise to skipped generations. Age at onset can vary widely within the same family.

144   Maternal serum alphafetoprotein (MSAFP) is found to be elevated above the 97th percentile (more than 2.5 multiples of the median) on a routine antenatal sample at 17 weeks gestation.
   a   What are the causes of elevated MSAFP?
   b   What is the subsequent management?

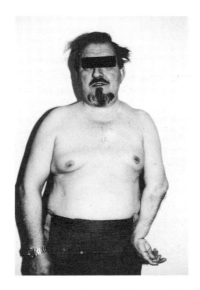

145   This man has non-progressive spastic paraplegia.
   a   What abnormalities are shown?
   b   What is the likely diagnosis?
   c   What is the recurrence risk?

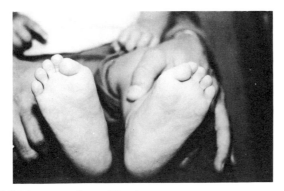

146   This child has ectopic ossification.
   a   What is the diagnosis?
   b   What is the prognosis?
   c   What is the mode of inheritance?

144 Maternal serum alphafetoprotein
a The causes of elevated MSAFP can be divided into two groups.
  1 With normal amniotic fluid AFP: normal finding (result in the top 3% of the distribution); wrong dates; twins; threatened abortion; maternal hereditary persistence of AFP.
  2 With elevated amniotic fluid AFP: anencephaly; open spina bifida; anterior abdominal wall defect; fetal teratoma; congenital nephrotic syndrome; fetal skin defects and placental haemangioma.
b The MSAFP should be repeated and ultrasound examination performed to check the gestation, exclude twins and look for neural tube defects and other abnormalities. If ultrasound examination does not provide an explanation but the second MSAFP is elevated, amniocentesis is indicated for measurement of amniotic fluid AFP and acetylcholinesterase banding. If this gives an abnormal result, further detailed ultrasound examination should be carried out.

145 Birth injury
a His left arm is smaller than the right and is held in the classic waiter's tip position.
b His arm abnormalities are due to a brachial plexus injury (Erbs palsy) and the association with non-progressive spastic paraplegia suggests birth injury as the cause of his problems.
c The recurrence risk for birth injury is not increased above the general population incidence.

146 Progressive myositis ossificans
a Short deviated big toes with a single phalanx and ectopic ossification are pathognomonic of progressive myositis ossificans (fibrodysplasia ossificans progressiva).
b Progressive physical handicap is invariable due to joint ankylosis with ectopic bone.
c Autosomal dominant with most patients resulting from new mutations.

147   A woman requests genetic counselling prior to embarking on her
      first pregnancy as her two brothers have severe haemophilia A.
      Her level of factor VIII coagulant activity is 130%.
      a   What is her pedigree risk of being a carrier for haemophilia A?
      b   Does her factor VIII level alter her carrier risk?

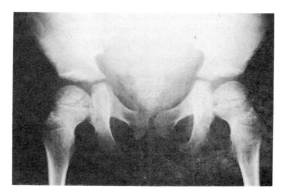

148   This is the X-ray of the pelvis of a teenager with trisomy 21.
      a   What complication is suggested?
      b   How would this be confirmed?

149   A twelve-year-old girl is investigated for non-progressive severe
      mental retardation unassociated with other physical
      abnormalities. There was no exposure to noxious agents during
      pregnancy, the delivery was normal at term and an earlier screen
      for fetal infection was negative. Urine mucopolysaccharides are
      not increased. Blood and urine amino acids and organic acids are
      normal. Chromosome analysis shows a normal female karyotype
      with no evidence of fragile X in folate deficient medium. Parents
      are healthy and unrelated and there is no other family history.
      a   What is the likely diagnosis?
      b   What is the recurrence risk?

147 Haemophilia A

a Haemophilia A is an X-linked recessive trait. This woman has a 1 in 2 pedigree risk of being a carrier since her mother with two affected sons is an obligate carrier.

b Factor VIII coagulant activity (factor VIIIc) varies in normal women from 50–150%. In 25–50% of carriers for haemophilia A the level of factor VIIIc is abnormally low but in the remainder values are within the normal range. Factor VIII can also be assayed immunologically (factor VIIIAg). In normal women there is usually good correlation between VIIIc and VIIIAg levels whereas in carriers the factor VIIIc level is often much lower than the factor VIIIAg. By comparing the two values 70–94% of carriers in haemophilia A families can be detected. The gene for factor VIII has recently been isolated and carrier detection using intragenic restriction fragment length polymorphisms (RFLPs) is likely to become the procedure of choice for carrier detection. The molecular approach also permits first trimester prenatal diagnosis whereas previously fetal blood sampling was required in at risk male pregnancies.

148 Trisomy 21 with hypothyroidism

a Hypothyroidism is not infrequent in trisomy 21 and is suggested by the fragmented capital femoral epiphyses.

b Serum T_4 will be low and TSH elevated.

149 Non-specific mental retardation

a In approximately one half of children investigated for moderate and severe mental retardation no cause can be identified. This is referred to as non-specific mental retardation and is likely to be a heterogeneous group.

b The empiric recurrence risk for a further affected child in this family is about 1 in 30. This risk is obtained by studying large numbers of families at risk. If the proband had been male the risk would have been higher because of as yet undelineated causes of X-linked mental retardation.

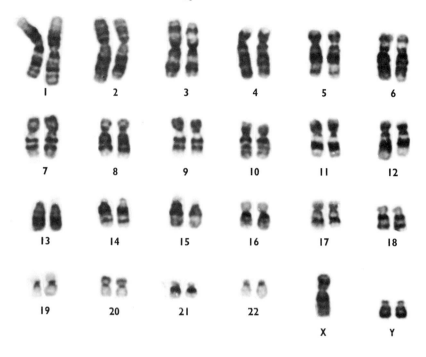

150 A 40-year-old woman has an amniocentesis in view of her age.
The fetal karyotype is shown above.
a What abnormality is present?
b What is the prognosis?

151 A healthy young couple request counselling because the man's
mother has been diagnosed as having polycystic kidney disease.
a How is this condition inherited?
b Can this man be reassured that he has not inherited the gene
for this disorder?
c What is the prognosis for individuals with this condition?

150   47, XYY

a   There is an extra Y chromosome present giving the karyotype 47, XYY.

b   The prevalence of 47, XYY is 1 per 1000 males in the general population as compared to nearly 1% in prisons and high security mental institutions. Nevertheless most 47, XYY individuals lead normal lives and the association with aggresive criminal behaviour has been over-emphasized. Prospective studies of cases ascertained by newborn screening have shown that most 47, XYY children are normal in appearance and intellectual development. There is a skew to the left in IQ distribution but this is small. Whilst some parents decide to continue with such a pregnancy, others will request termination.

151   Adult polycystic kidney disease

a   Autosomal dominant with variable age of onset. The offspring of an affected individual have a 1 in 2 chance of inheriting the disease gene, but if they remain healthy the risk that they are carriers will steadily fall through adult life, becoming very low beyond the age of 65.

b   No. Symptoms are rare in childhood and 85% of gene carriers under 30 years of age are symptom free. This man needs a physical examination to exclude hypertension and palpable kidney enlargement, routine testing and culture of his urine and renal ultrasound. In one large study radionuclide imaging and pyelography with tomography were both superior to ultrasound in identifying carriers by detecting renal cysts, but with recent improvements in ultrasound imaging this may no longer be the case. These methods will identify the majority of asymptomatic gene carriers over the age of 20 and if no abnormality is detected the risk is probably less than 5%. The role of computerized axial tomography has not been established. Recent evidence suggests that the locus for this disorder is on chromosome 16 and linked probes should be useful aids for genetic counselling.

c   Renal failure is the eventual outcome in most cases. It is hoped that the prognosis can be improved with the early detection of affected individuals by family screening so that complications such as hypertension and urinary tract infections can be treated promptly.

152   **A couple request counselling because their first child has**
         arthrogryposis multiplex congenita.
         a What is the cause of this condition?
         b What is the recurrence risk?
         c Is prenatal diagnosis available?

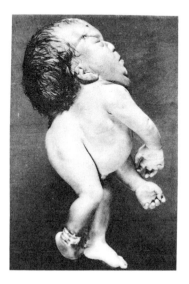

153   **a** What is the abnormality shown?
         b What is the recurrence risk?

152   Arthrogryposis

a   The term arthrogryposis multiplex congenita describes
    congenital contractures affecting several joints and does not in
    itself constitute a diagnosis. There are many causes including
    oligohydramnios, maternal myasthenia gravis, congenital
    myotonic dystrophy and other myopathies, trisomy 18, neural
    tube defect and idiopathic anterior horn cell loss.
    Arthrogryposis occurs as part of the autosomal recessive
    Pena-Shokeir syndrome and there are several types of
    autosomal dominant distal arthrogryposis. Clearly it is essential
    to take a full family history and carry out a careful examination
    and investigations to determine if the arthrogryposis has a
    myopathic or neurogenic aetiology or forms part of an inherited
    syndrome.

b   If no specific cause can be identified and there is no family
    history the recurrence risk is low. When the index case is not
    available for investigation the empiric recurrence risk is around
    5% (10% in cases associated with neonatal death).

c   Except for the few cases associated with a chromosome
    abnormality, neural tube defect or myotonic dystrophy, prenatal
    diagnosis is unsatisfactory. Occasionally joint limitation may be
    apparent on an ultrasound scan.

153   Iniencephaly

a   The head is large compared to the trunk and the upper spine is
    hyperextended so that the face looks upward. The neck is all but
    eliminated. This severe malformation, which is incompatible
    with prolonged extrauterine life, is called iniencephaly.
    Additional CNS and other abnormalities are often present.

b   This is a rare abnormality and the recurrence risk is not known
    but iniencephaly is usually regarded as part of the neural tube
    defect spectrum and prenatal diagnosis by ultrasound scanning
    and amniocentesis is recommended.

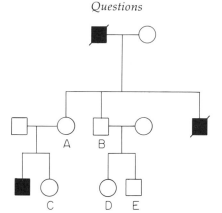

154 **This is a family with hypertrophic obstructive cardiomyopathy
     (HOCM). Symptomatic individuals are shaded.**
   a What is the mode of transmission in this family?
   b Which members of the family are at negligible risk of carrying
       the gene for HOCM?
   c What investigations are indicated?
   d What is the prognosis for individuals who inherit the disease
       gene?

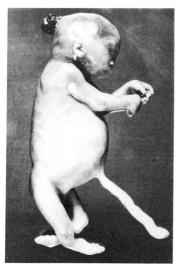

155 **This newborn has polydactyly.**
   a What is the diagnosis?
   b What other features may be present?
   c What is the recurrence risk?
   d Is prenatal diagnosis available?

154   Hypertrophic obstructive cardiomyopathy (HOCM)

   a HOCM usually shows autosomal dominant transmission and this family would be consistent with this mode of inheritance. By chance only males have been affected but male to male transmission rules out X-linked recessive inheritance. In this condition expression is very variable and only 25% of carriers of the disease gene are symptomatic. An example is individual A who is unaffected but must carry the gene since she has transmitted it to her son.

   b None. B and C had a 1 in 2 chance of inheriting the disease gene at conception and the fact that they are asymptomatic only results in a small reduction in this risk (from 50% to about 43%). For D and E the risk is far from negligible (being about 17%).

   c Characteristic echocardiographic abnormalities including asymmetrical ventricular septal hypertrophy can be demonstrated in most individuals who carry the HOCM gene. Echocardiography is therefore an essential prerequisite to risk estimation and genetic counselling.

   d The prognosis is extraordinarily variable. Symptoms can develop at any age and include fatigue, dyspnoea with exercise, palpitations, angina pectoris and syncope. Beta blockers may be effective. There is a risk of sudden death even in childhood. In contrast, about 75% of individuals who carry the gene are asymptomatic and have a normal life span.

155   Meckel syndrome

   a The combination of occipital encephalocele, micrognathia, polydactyly and abdominal distension suggests the Meckel syndrome.

   b The abdominal distension is due to very large cystic dysplastic kidneys. Other features include microphthalmia, cleft palate and incomplete development of external genitalia.

   c This is an autosomal recessive disorder with a 1 in 4 recurrence risk.

   d Prenatal diagnosis is possible with ultrasound by detection of the encephalocele, polydactyly or renal cysts.

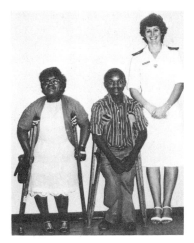

156 **This mother and her son have rickets.**
   a What inherited disorder should be considered?
   b How may this be confirmed?
   c What is the mode of inheritance?

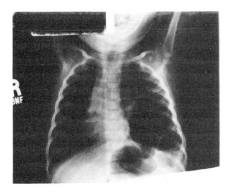

157 **This neonate has respiratory distress.**
   a What is the diagnosis?
   b What is the recurrence risk?
   c Is prenatal diagnosis possible?

156   Vitamin D-resistant rickets
  a   The mother and son have marked short stature and rickets.
      Whilst this could be dietary an inherited type of rickets is
      suggested and with transmission from mother to offspring
      vitamin D-resistant rickets is likely.
  b   Serum phosphate is reduced, hence the alternative name
      Familial Hypophosphataemic Rickets.
  c   This is an X-linked dominant disorder. Half of the offspring
      (male and female) of an affected woman will be affected whilst
      for an affected man all his daughters will be affected but all his
      sons will be normal (an important distinguishing feature from
      autosomal dominant inheritance).

157   a   Diaphragmatic hernia.
  b   The frequency of congenital diaphragmatic hernia is about 1 per
      2000 total births. In most families it appears to be sporadic with
      a low recurrence risk but there have been a few reports of more
      than one affected child in a family.
  c   A large defect can be demonstrated with ultrasound.

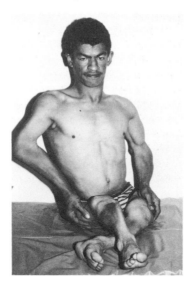

158 **This man has blue sclerae. His mother also has blue sclerae but no other abnormalities.**
   a What is the diagnosis?
   b What other physical findings may be present in this man?
   c Does the mother have the same condition?
   d What is the aetiology?

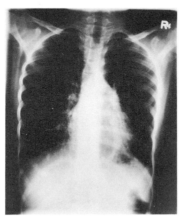

159 **This is the chest X-ray of a 12-year-old girl with recurrent chest and sinus infections.**
   a What is the diagnosis?
   b What other features may occur in this condition?
   c What is the mode of inheritance?

158 Osteogenesis imperfecta

a Blue sclerae and deformities of the upper and lower limbs due to multiple fractures are features of osteogenesis imperfecta (OI).

b Deafness due to otosclerosis, discoloured teeth (dentinogenesis imperfecta), lax joints and hernias.

c The majority of adult cases of OI are autosomal dominant. Expression can be extraordinarily variable within the same family, some individuals being severely handicapped and others having blue sclerae as the only manifestation, as in this example. Before concluding that an apparently sporadic case represents a new mutation it is essential to examine the parents and other close relatives.

d Biochemical and molecular studies indicate that OI is not one but multiple different conditions (genetic heterogeneity) each of which represents a fault in the production of collagen.

159 Kartagener's syndrome

a The combination of recurrent chest and sinus infections with total situs inversus is typical of Kartagener's syndrome.

b Congenital heart disease may be present. Infertility due to defective sperm motility is usual in males. Sperm tails and respiratory cilia lack dynein which is important for normal motility.

c Inheritance is thought to be autosomal recessive, but there appears to be incomplete penetrance so that the recurrence risk in siblings is less than the expected 25%.

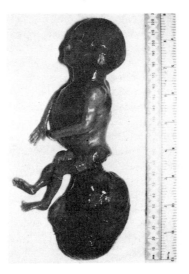

160 **a** What is the likely diagnosis?
   b What is the prognosis?
   c What is the recurrence risk?
   d Is prenatal diagnosis possible?

160 Sacrococcygeal teratoma
  a The differential diagnosis of this sacral mass includes a
    myelomeningocele, a sacrococcygeal teratoma and other rarer
    tumours such as neuroblastoma, chordoma or papillary
    ependymoma. A myelomeningocele can be clinically excluded
    but biopsy is required to confirm the tumour pathology.
  b Most sacrococcygeal teratomas are benign and surgically
    curable.
  c The recurrence risk is negligible.
  d Elevated MSAFP may occur and the mass can be visualized
    with ultrasound.

Glossary

Alleles alternative forms of a gene at the same locus

Amniocentesis aspiration of amniotic fluid

Aneuploid any chromosome number which is not an exact multiple of the haploid number

Ascertainment identification of families with an inherited condition

Autosome any chromosome other than the sex chromosomes

Burden consultand's perception of the cost (emotional, physical and financial) of a genetic disorder

Carrier a recessive heterozygote

Chimaera an individual whose cells are derived from more than one zygote

Clone a cell line derived by mitosis from a single diploid cell

Codominant both alleles of a pair are expressed in the heterozygote

Codon three adjacent bases in DNA or RNA which specify an aminoacid

Compound an individual with two different mutant alleles at a locus on homologous chromosomes

Concordant both members of a twin pair show the trait

Congenital present at birth

Consanguineous mating between individuals who share at least one common ancestor

Consultand any person requesting genetic counselling

Crossover exchange of genetic material between homologous chromosomes during meiosis

Diploid the chromosome number of somatic cells

Discordant only one member of a twin pair shows the trait

Dominant a trait expressed in the heterozygote

Empiric risk recurrence risk based on experience rather than calculation

Exon a coding region of a gene

Fetoscopy endoscopic visualization of the fetus

Forme fruste an incomplete, partial or mild form of a trait or syndrome

Gene a sequence of bases in DNA which codes for one polypeptide

Genetic counselling the communication of information and advice about inherited disorders

Genetic engineering the artificial production of new combinations of heritable material

Genetic lethal a genetic disorder in which affected individuals fail to reproduce

Genome the genetic constitution of an individual

Genotype the alleles present at one locus

Hemizygous genes on the X chromosome in males

Heredity   the transmission of characteristics to descendents
Heterogeneity   similar phenotypes from different genotypes
Heterozygote   an individual with one normal and one mutant allele at a given locus on a pair of homologous chromosomes
Homologous   matched
Homozygote   an individual with a pair of identical alleles at a given locus on homologous chromosomes
Idiogram   a diagram of the chromosome complement
Inbreeding   the mating of closely related individuals
Intron   a non-coding region of a gene
Isochromosome   an abnormal chromosome with duplication of one arm and deletion of the other caused by transverse division of the centromere
Karyotype   the classified chromosome complement of an individual or cell
Kindred   an extended family
Linkage   linked genes have their loci within measurable distance of one another on the same chromosome
Locus   the precise location of a gene on a chromosome
Meiosis   reduction cell division which occurs in gamete production
Mitosis   somatic cell division
Monosomy   one of a chromosome pair is missing
Mosaic   an individual derived from a single zygote with cells of two or more different genotypes
Multifactorial   inheritance due to multiple genes at different loci which summate and interact with environmental factors
Mutation   a change in the genetic material
Nondisjunction   failure of two members of a chromosome pair to disjoin during anaphase
Nucleotide   a purine or pyrimidine base attached to a sugar and phosphate group
Oncogene   a gene sequence capable of causing transformation
Penetrance   the frequency of expression of the genotype
Phenocopy   an environmentally induced mimic of a genetic disease
Phenotype   the observable characteristics of an individual
Pleiotropy   multiple effects of a single gene
Polygenic   determined by multiple genes at different loci each with a small but additive effect
Polymorphism   the occurrence together in a population of two or more discontinuous traits in such proportions that the frequency of the rarest could not be maintained only by recurrent mutation.
Polyploid   an abnormal chromosomal complement which exceeds the diploid number and is an exact multiple of the haploid number
Proband   the individual who draws medical attention to the family
Probe   a radiolabelled DNA fragment used to identify a complementary sequence(s)

Recessive a trait which is expressed only in homozygotes

Recombinant an individual in a linkage study in whom the marker and disease loci have assorted at parental meiosis

Recombinant DNA artificial insertion of a portion of DNA from one organism into the genome of another

Recombination the formation of new combinations of linked genes by crossing over between their loci during meiosis

Restriction enzyme an enzyme which cleaves DNA at sequence specific sites (the recognition site)

Restriction fragment length polymorphism (RFLP) a recognition site for a restriction enzyme which may or may not be present

Segregation the separation of allelic genes at meiosis

Sex-limited a trait expressed only in one sex

Sex-linked inheritance of a gene carried on a sex chromosome

Sporadic no known genetic basis

Teratogen any agent which causes congenital malformations

Trait any gene determined characteristic

Translation conversion of the mRNA message to a polypeptide chain

Translocation the transfer of chromosomal material between chromosomes

Triploid a cell with three times the haploid number of chromosomes

Trisomy three copies of a given chromosome per cell

Zygote the fertilized ovum

Further Reading

Basic genetics
Goodenough U. (1984) *Genetics*, 3rd ed. Saunders College Publishing, Philadelphia.
Old R.W. & Primrose S.B. (1985) *Principles of Gene Manipulation*, 3rd ed. Blackwell Scientific Publications, Oxford.

Clinical molecular genetics
Emery A.E.H. (1984) *An Introduction to Recombinant DNA*. John Wiley & Sons, Chichester.
Weatherall D.J. (1985) *The New Genetics and Clinical Practice* 2nd ed. Nuffield Provincial Hospitals Trust, London.

Genetic counselling
Connor J.M. & Ferguson-Smith M.A. (1984) *Essential Medical Genetics*. Blackwell Scientific Publications, Oxford.
Emery A.E.H. (1976) *Methodology in Medical Genetics*. Churchill Livingstone, Edinburgh.
Harper P.S. (1984) *Practical Genetic Counselling*, 2nd ed. John Wright & Sons, Bristol.

Syndrome identification
Baraitser M. & Winter R. (1983) *A Colour Atlas of Clinical Genetics*. Wolfe Medical Publications, London.
Gorlin R.J., Pinborg J.J. & Cohen M.M. (1976) *Syndromes of the Head and Neck*, 2nd ed. McGraw-Hill, New York.
Holmes L.B., Moser H.W., Halldórsson S., Mack C., Pant S.S. & Matzilevich B. (1972) *Mental Retardation. An Atlas of Diseases with Associated Physical Abnormalities*. Macmillan Publishing Co., New York
Smith D.W. (1982) *Recognisable Patterns of Human Malformation*, 3rd ed. W.B. Saunders, New York.

Further information about particular genetic diseases
Baraitser M. (1982) *The Genetics of Neurological Disorders*. Oxford University Press, Oxford.
Beighton P. (1978) *Inherited Disorders of the Skeleton*. Churchill Livingstone, Edinburgh.
Bergsma D.S. (1979) *Birth Defects Atlas and Compendium*, 2nd ed. Williams & Wilkins, Baltimore.
Bundey S. (1985) *Genetics and Neurology*. Churchill Livingstone, Edinburgh.

Emery A.E.H. & Rimoin D.L. (1983) *The Principles and Practice of Medical Genetics*. Churchill Livingstone, Edinburgh.

der Kaloustian V.M. & Kuorban A.K. (1979) *Genetic Diseases of the Skin*. Springer-Verlag, Berlin.

Keith C.G. (1978) *Genetics and Ophthalmology*. Churchill Livingstone, Edinburgh.

Koningsmark B.W. & Gorlin R.J. (1976) *Genetic and Metabolic Deafness* W.B. Saunders, Philadelphia.

McKusick V.A. (1984) *Mendelian Inheritance in Man: Catalogs of Autosomal Dominant, Autosomal Recessive and X-linked Phenotypes*, 6th ed. The John Hopkins Press, Baltimore.

Spranger J., Langer L.O. & Wiedemann H.R. (1974) *Bone Dysplasias. An Atlas of Constitutional Disorders of Skeletal Development*. Gustav Fischer Verlag, Stuttgart.

Stanbury J.B., Wyngaarden J.B., Fredrickson D.S. & Goldstein J.L. (1983) *The Metabolic Basis of Inherited Disease*, 5th ed. McGraw-Hill, New York.

Warkany J. (1971) *Congenital Malformations*. Year Book Medical Publishers, Chicago.

Index

Entries refer to question numbers